A Stranger's Heart:
Poems by a Critical Care Physician

Phillip J. Cozzi

Acknowledgements:

The author wishes to thank the editors of the following publications in which poems previously appeared: "The Fabric Anthology of Green" in *Rhino*, "Empathy for an Orange," which received the Morton Marr Poetry Prize from *The Southwest Review*, "Hong Kong Crane" in *The Eloquent Poem* edited by Elise Paschen published by Persea Press, "First Clinic Visit with Mr. Schrammel" in *The New England Journal of Medicine*, "Clinic Chart" in *The Journal of the American Medical Association*, "Overdose by Ingestion," "Fellows," "Dr. Thommes and Dr. Woods," "On Viewing The Anatomy Lesson," "Ode," "Cardiac Silhouette Seen On Chest X-ray," Stranger's Heart," "Sonnet ForShirley," "Popsicle," "Concerning Emma" (which won the inaugural Annual Poetry Prize from the American College of Physicians), "Voices of the ICU" and "Apple Core Lesion" in *The Annals of Internal Medicine*, and "Love Poem of the Rural Doc" in *The Western Journal of Medicine*.

For Dar, the love of my life
For my parents, Paul and Eileen

TABLE OF CONTENTS

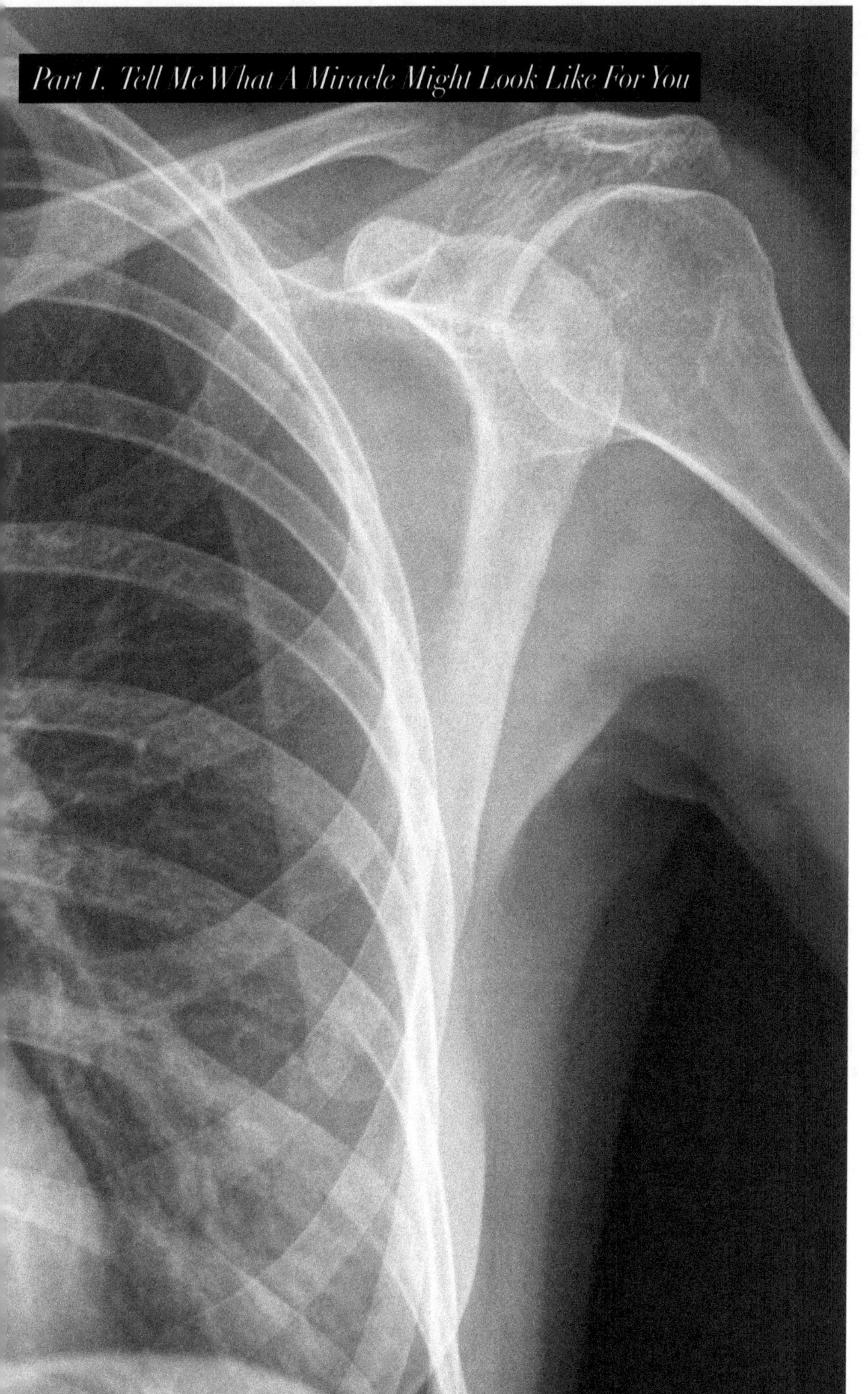
Part I. Tell Me What A Miracle Might Look Like For You

THE FABRIC ANTHOLOGY OF GREEN

Close your eyes and read with fingertip the fabric anthology of green, pledgets
bound by Amy, cut from curtain and sweater, napkin and day dress, surgical linen
beginning with the Robin Hood Halloween costume green, the flower stem green,
the Aunt Norma green, the Indian Ocean, tortoise back, Girl Scout green,

then turn the page to the sun-washed gun-metal green glinting off tanks
as they ground the rubble of St. Petersburg, Sorrento, Fussen, moss drenching
viaduct under which you parked your bike and dreamed of Cindy Tonelli,
avocado of the mind, seeded and sold cold by the bushel on California highways,

green apply jelly bean, bok choy, olive, gallstone, bile, kiwi, the tree weeping
like a child, the paisley upholstery petrified in Uncle Joe's living room, verdigris
eating Lincoln's profile, the relief map continent of South America as you
palpate the Andes' peaks, sycamore veins and the spiky Komodo,

the green-glazed bricks of magic animals in relief on the Temple of Morduk,
the almost-black green of Rembrandt depicting Aristotle contemplating Homer,
the foothills of childhood, umbrella pine, Burma, cobalt, ground laurel,
the clippings of cubist art on the floor of Ed Toczylowski's Florist Shop,

tongue of glacier blanketing Greenland, as green with envy, nausea, naiveté,
green encroaching like lichen on log, until all the Earth is green, all is green
as with the phosgene spark which started it all, captured and carried with poles
and buried with the Ark of the Covenant, with a pot of manna and stone tablets,

to emerge holy in emerald anarchy signifying Spring, as in the first moment
of the very first season: the green of wild grain at the dawn of human life.

 Phillip J. Cozzi

LANGUAGE LINE

Because this is a love poem, you
don't expect words like Pseudomonas,
calvarium, *edema,* encephalopathy
to scamper on scorpion legs across the page,
nor the lovely *aeruginosa* to hover
as nervous laughter, cloud of gnats.
Nor should you expect the babble
of moisture in ventilator tubing,
the trickling language of urine.

But trust me, when a rainy night
veers toward the curb and skids,
there is no love so azure
and because you long to understand
love without limits, not the satisfying,
help-me-be-my-best-self
floral print kind of love, you phone
the language line with Juan's mother.

Juan stepped out of a bar on Cermak Road
into traffic. When his skull was removed
to allow his brain to swell,
his head looked shark-bitten.
When cerebrospinal fluid churned
and burbled from cracks deep within,
his head swelled massively. His mother
wants you to keep him alive.
On the hospital end table, a photo
of Juan cradling his infant son
shows the shapes of their heads
were once identical,
thick black turf covering each.

The word *craniectomy* has Latin roots
but no English-Spanish dictionary dries
this pressed flower, forgotten blue agave.
The word *limits* has red-yellow stripes,

a triangular head, only one of four
venomous species known to the Yucatan.
You release the wire cage door.
The word rouses
then the flash of fang.

And what happens, you might ask,
when you advise limits? Foreign syllables
start reaching one for the next. A faceless
interpreter on speaker phone summons images
of a woman building an altar of water.
You hear in her voice a wall of rain,
the dialogue of sheets, an eddy of language
swirling first in the corner of the room
then gaining speed, words chasing each other,
while the bed lifts like the Pequod,
the floor-swell heaves and falls,
tongue clicks as latches of a storm door being
ripped free, before the bone-shaking howl,
the typhoon eye, and you,
lashed to the mast of a cell phone,
learn love translates to something carnal,
a drowning, a catastrophic craving.

 Phillip J. Cozzi

WHAT TO BRING TO THE ICU FAMILY CONFERENCE

Falling snow
A goldfish in a plastic bag
Larkspur and bluebunch wheatgrass
The cakewalk from Mission Day
And when each of Bernice's nine daughters
    start bristling with hatred for each other, bring out
A lagoon
The trail of cedars
Human weakness, sleeping
Rosehips
The dozing of the caterpillar
Fig preserves
Ithaca, Greece
Prairie light
A foal
Fretted, frayed rope
A kitchenette
Prehensile tails
The essence of regret
Rain pouring from gutters
An ostrich feather
The music of Otis Redding
Mint leaf
A small lawn which needs mowing
A red bouncy ball
Pawprint of black bear
Carrier Pigeon
The meagerness of reason
Snap pea, ginger snaps and licorice snaps
Gertrude Stein
A nest
St. Jerome
The Niagara Falls
A few minutes of small round stones
And you must bring the words, "Bernice is dying," as well as
A snoring dog, leaning against the side of the house
An algae-covered starfish

Phillip J. Cozzi 11

Your faults
Five centuries
A whale-oil reading lamp
An old-style marquee
Silence
The Boxcar Children
Wedding dresses
You might forego the powder keg and loose fire ants
    but an ant farm may just do the trick
A silver maple
Shyness
A goose with head turned backward, beak tucked
    under wing feather
Hundreds of luminous jellyfish
Coffee can full of pennies and buttons
Cartwheel
The difficulty of language understood,
    not understood or resisted
The blue apples of Paul Cezanne
The crunch of the pear
And, of course, the memory of nine children
    in one bedroom
The list of plants at the Lurie Gardens
Collarbones.

PECULIAR

When I pry your eyes open
with my fingers, I see
the skin of a ripe plum breaking apart
or two widely-dilated circles
of friends sharing plum brandy
or the wine-bruised forearms
or doll's eyes fixed in your head
as if forever focused on a single
jaundiced thought, bile having risen
in bubbles from bowel to sclera
and my gaze turns to your wife,
delirious with sleep deprivation
from plastic night after night in ICU
and whom you continue to abuse,
with peculiar skill, even from your coma.

A RAPID RESPONSE, 4 AM

On a scale of 1 to 10
how delicate is the darkness
icy the lighting
silent the daughter
tender the union
stranger the poetry
intimate the thought
ancient the blood
secret the language
patient the patient
awaiting dissolution
of nitroglycerin
under tongue?
Their faces: Spanish
beautifully silvered
brushstrokes of moonlight.
Their souls: a flock
of birds leaving
a tree, then returning.

EMPATHY FOR AN ORANGE

I can't even imagine how painful this must be,
waiting in a bowl on the kitchen island, pensive
planet, thought-filled and enigmatic. Tell me
about your dad, or one memory of the bough
on which your mother cradled her fruit,
that seed-laden, world-weary, gracious bough.
You might be feeling alone, scared, frustrated
and this might come as a shock to you
but at least one person admires your strength,
your symmetry and innuendoes, your involvement
and inescapable rhythms, your animal eye
and embryonic imagination, philosophical pose,
statement on mathematics, chemical dreams.
You are funny and sensuous when peeled in a spiral,
made only more beautiful by dribbling down the chin
then wiped with the back of the hand. This helps me
better understand what you are thinking. Tell me
what a miracle might look like for you.

OVERDOSE BY INGESTION

The slender body measured toe to crown
is sixty inches long. The hair is brown
but light in front. A ponytail is wound
with soft cloth loops.

The eyes are closed. The mouth is open just
enough to see the teeth remain in place,
in fair repair. The ears are pierced
five times each.

The trachea is midline to the chest
which is without deformity. The breasts
are large in size, symmetrical except
for two paddle burns.

The abdomen is silent, soft and flat.
External genitalia: adult,
of female type. Extremities intact,
with nails cut short.

Between the feet, transparent plastic sacks
reveal the blouse and shoes. A pair of slacks
with flowered print is stuffed into a bag
and tangled with itself.

HOMAGE TO THE COLLARBONE

For framing Darlene's face above, the heart below.
For sharing the story of the ice-skating accident with a callus.
For bringing to mind, when bared, the slender s-shaped vents of the violin.
For bringing to life the scrolled embellishments on the chapel
	within the Arc de Triomphe.
For floating like water lily.
For opening like hand to rain.
For loveliness and loneliness.
For making elegant sexy, again and again.
For extending humility wherever turned.
For flying like a buttress, Gothic-style.
For pointing outward and inward.
For protecting the great vessels.
For asking so little.
For frightening Spanish schoolchildren: clavicula.
For suffering piercing and tattoo.
For strutting sternum to shoulder.
For lounging on an invisible chaise.
For being doubly curved.
For meaning in Latin "little key," rotating along its axis.
For appearing in the 5th week of gestation.
For running behind and below the gills of primitive bony fish.
	One day, Darlene chased our son Phillip on the ice
	at Ridgeland Commons Skating Rink. She tripped and, later,
	kept telling the ER staff that her husband is a physician,
	to find him, but nobody could find me.
For respecting solitude.
For making emptiness possible, with the twinned gullies
	of supraclavicular fossae.
For being the most commonly fractured bone.

Phillip J. Cozzi 17

THE ART OF THE SQUIRREL

is the art of hesitation. Fur
in rapid brushstrokes. Face
in delicate inkwork. Expression
in still-wet frescoed pigment. Mouth,
the opening of a kiln. Chest
in vaulted grandeur. Tail
in calligraphy. Line
portraying movement. Narrative
of acorn dream. Philosophy
of anonymous craftsman. Tone
of nutmeg lamentation. Gait
tentative as the seventh century
striding into written language. Sudden
statue of himself. Monument
to conquest of picnic table. Gaze
sweeps our yard like stained glass
swept through Europe, then fixes us,
etched into antiquity: blue
figures on this morning's vase.

 Phillip J. Cozzi

CONCH

Strange place for a conch
on the floor of a bathroom
in the suburbs of Chicago,
disquieting the home's visitors
and even the residents
who had forgotten its origins.

A memento from the Caribbean,
perhaps. A splash of life
from a burdened soul,
and to think a soul
once dwelled in this housing,
scuttled a different floor,

or that a soul lived
in every single shell
at one time, each onus
becoming more beautiful,
to be discovered by a child,
a marvel to behold, an elegant

pink and khaki spiny spiral.
Triton's trumpet. At one time
every boat bore a conch
to send a baleful note across
the wide-open waters
of humanity. This animal

is an unsettling argument.
Prized by sun-browned divers
for bringing fertility,
the meat is mallet-pounded,
sautéed and slurped down
at The Feast of Seven Fishes

on Christmas Eve. So often,
death is the harbinger
of birth. *Scungilli,* in Italian,

the bastard child of the original
Sanskrit word *sankha,* somehow
devolved to conch.

But conch is the best name
for this floor-dwelling hermit,
displaced and disconcerting,
like dangerous reasoning
with a point at both ends.

 Phillip J. Cozzi

THE ROLE OF THE COMMA

For Catherine Downes

When my husband and I separated,
I thought about the comma,
that chubby single-tailed protozoan,

Haley's comet, lure and fishhook,
one-legged pregnant lady, lost eyebrow.
When my husband and I separated

I thought of the role of the comma
in separating the elements of a series
such as "You, I, your grad-student girlfriend"

and how it is all but mandatory
in formal writing, as omission brings ambiguity.
He always said I never understood

the role of the comma, as in "Naturally,
I agree with you." or "Last summer,
you went on a long vacation."

Tiny cat-scratch punctuation,
microscopic wound and valediction
as even now I confess to never

having mastered making lunches, making beds,
or the use of that sperm-shaped ink-blot,
that often-unnecessary flagellated planet.

True, he was deft with the comma
in writing the aside, such as, "We have,
in a manner of speaking, won despite our loss."

I lost the single-feathered dream catcher,
wind-blown wind chime, winking eye, embryo,
cashew, croissant, crescent moon,
tadpole, talon, grammatical eyelash.

SKATING BACKWARDS

What's important here is what's not here:
a physical reminiscence of pushing away,

keeping the blades straight, then working the heels
apart and together to swizzle back years

from wellness to cancer to wellness, the reverse
wedding, the reappearance of Joe Beaumont

who died as a boy, weaving through grades 12 to 1,
even centuries back to a frozen canal,

the salted taste of wintered lips, the scrub
of fierce wind, the indifference of ice,

while trying to keep the hips beneath oneself
which, as you know, can be hard to do,

turning in ancient spiritual tradition
by shifting your weight from foot to foot,

frost stiffened cuffs, slapface cold, the edges
etching in disappearing Dutch, the humility

of an awkward climb back onto feet
to balance grace and landscape, life

gliding forward, backwards and blindly,
an exhilarating view of where you have been.

 Phillip J. Cozzi

PAPER MACHE SPHINX

Newsprint runs backwards to 1969
and weaves in black block letters. A headline
with the words U.S. and TROOPS is cut
into strips, soaked in a water and flour slurry,
but you have to read backwards
through the thin translucent paper
as some strips lie face down
with design reversed. The story is lost
somewhere in the torso. You can imagine
a diligent fourth-grader running
his soft hand head to rump
to smooth the edges, a mother stirring
a pot on a stove, and a father
with an unlit stump of a cigar
in the corner of his mouth
marveling at the newborn creature
ancient on his kitchen table.
A pride in a school project:
head of man, body of lion
while the boy's hand palpates
a faintly bleating, mythological heart,
an oracle, a talisman keeping the draft
out of the home. If only they knew
the right questions to ask
the sage. Brushed with glue,
then drizzled with sand, the god
was carried on cardboard in the child's arms,
a stately procession down the alleys
of south Oak Park to Ascension Grammar School,
where classmates ogled the deity
before it returned home in a bag. And
although that boy tries and tries
to finish his poems on a happy note,
he now sees a man named Clement, in the ER,
who chose to shoot himself in the face
which reminds the boy of the Great Sphinx
of Giza whose nose was defaced
by vandals, hundreds of years ago.

THE GAME OF SCENT

It's your turn. To smell the morning
before the first demanding sniff of work.

To shuffle in pj's through the citrus
of the kitchen out the back door.

To inhale the quirky promise of pine
the generosity of the sky.

To catch the complex fragrance
of fresh wind carrying floral

bounty bewitching acrobatic bees
this moment a whiff

pointedly impractical, sacred among senses
an animal involvement, a literature

luxurious and ascetic. To filter out distractions
and focus on each sun-mottled scent.

Yesterday, a man in robes encircled
Angie's coffin with incense

you learned was made of crushed hearts
of rose delivered from the Holy Land

but this morning has the scent of possibility
so you spin the pinwheel

of aroma, a zero-sum game,
a trembling hand perfection, impossible to win,

impossible to not win.

 Phillip J. Cozzi

THE MATHEMATICS OF ZSA ZSA GABOR

6,000,000, concentration camp prisoners in 1941,
 the year she escaped Nazi-occupied Hungary
3,300,000, paid to Elke Sommer in libel suit
215,000, cost of Rolls Royce
12,937, fines for slapping police officer
9,000, square-foot Hollywood Regency-style home in Bel-Air
1936, year crowned Miss Hungary
120, hours community service sentenced
100, mourners attended funeral
99, years of life
50, days shy of becoming a centenarian
30, movies
10, adopted children, all male
9, husbands
8, Johnny Carson appearances
4, doctors tried to save her leg
3, days in jail
2, Jewish parents
1, daughter, resulting from rape
0, breaths, urge to recall moments of shame
-1, right leg, tyrant, seductress, mother to 11, American amputee
-6,000,000, incinerated bodies,
    whose soot snowed black over Budapest and Győr
-24,000,000, Hungarian souls, with whom she reunited
     in a blinding camera flash, arms outstretched,
       the trademark "Dahlink" echoing toward infinity.

Part II. Her Torso Extends Like Long Lines of Poetry

THE MANY USES OF POETRY

Dear Matthew, I knew you wouldn't mind
if I used your latest volume
to keep the billiard table level. This way
all the balls don't rush toward one pocket.
And since I am striving to strangeify,
I have also used it as an oven mitt,
headrest, and even stand on it
to try to make myself taller, confounded
by the need to simultaneously wear the book
atop my head as a level
to mark my growth as a writer
on the door jam. And since the spirit
of the book has already entered me
like a big bowl of buttered noodles,
each scrumptious syllable intercalating
my deoxynucleics, why not make
a paper airplane of the table of contents?
A pirate hat of p. 91? I tore out
your bio, scrolled it into a telescope,
startled my wife with a gravelly "Ahoy!"
scanned the horizon for booty:
a bucket of defining characteristics
and the high dive of our youth.
Baking parchment. You rescued my family
when I couldn't light wet logs
on our soggy Kettle Moraine camping trip.

What wonderful kindling you make!
And since I have done none of these things
and all of these things, and owe you so much,
I invite you over to meet my family,
the one you saved, Darlene, Phillip,
Joseph, even Pickles the cat.
We will serve casserole on your book
become trivet, then you and I will head
to the basement for ceremonial commiseration
of failures over a quick game of pool.

SOUNDS WE MAKE WHEN ALONE

Thrumming fingers is *Rain Pelting Roof*.
Tapping hard shoe on hollow metal desk leg
is P*eal of Church Bells*. Thinking of Elizabeth
sounds *The Crackle of Neon*. *Clearing of the throat*
is heard as *Punching Bag Frenzy*, while clearing
of the mind is *I Surrender to the Violets*.
Nearly inaudible hum of background brainwave
is *Geese That Surpasseth Understanding*. When
thought turns to work, that is *Whoosh of Traffic*
but when work turns to thought that is
Truck Double Clutching. The flip of a journal page
is *Wingbeat of White Heron*, while multiple pages
is *Crunch of Boneyard Underfoot*. Occasionally,
Lightening Crack in the clicking of a ballpoint
is followed by *Scratch of Cat Claw*, then *Thud
of Bedroom Door*. Rubbing the face
with both hands is *Helicopter Approaching*.
A sigh becomes *The Drawing of a Cutlass*,
that distinct note of blade leaving sheath,
while preparing to swing on ropes over the bow
to claim booty for the night's fun: *Squeak
of Canvas Shoes, Auto Engine Awakening*
and each blink of the eye sounds out
Smooching on the Sidewalk. Imaginings,
Hiss of Locomotive Steam, and a shift of chair
becomes *Endlessly Revolving Hotel Doors* and
When a Child Questions an Adult's Choices.

 Phillip J. Cozzi

THROUGH THE GALLERY WINDOW

My wife and I study through glass
the bare backside of a woman
trying to figure out if she's real.
Photograph or painting? Wrunkled skin
of her feet: unspeakable. Texture
of hair, like the bark of Scottish pine,
is so hairlike as to frustrate,
a unifying idea just out of grasp.
She has turned her back to the street,
lies on her left side, arms over her head,
mooning the world, artfully. But wait,
we return the next day, crossing traffic
for something yet to be discovered:
her refusal to follow domestic life
and the unknowable lyric of her lumbar spine.
Length of her torso extends like long lines
o f poetry almost to the right margin.
Paired dimples in her shoulder blades
are no mere ornamental flourish,
but something we will never understand,
the beautiful evanescence of frost. Light
seeks out her flesh as if shaping sly discourse.
Profile of hip singes an orange line: forest fire
cresting the Santa Lucia range
at nightfall in Carmel, encroaching our rental.
We awaken to light spruce ash dusting the morning
and the clarity of knowing we'll never know.

READING GLASSES

All print was a smudge. The particulars
were particularly misty to my has-been
eyeballs, which is why my ex-sister-in-law Vivian
gave me her reading glasses for which I grope
in the dark at the bedside table.
These readers have been through a lot,
first sported by her ex-husband, Rick,
of whose whereabouts nobody knows,
then dumped by Vi, whose vision
demanded something more stylish,
then gifted to me, a symbol of decrepitude,
which could have belonged to a British spy,
considering the impression they leave.
Grey, square, tortoise-shelled, too like me
to tolerate. One loose earpiece rides
at an angle, so that one eye appears
freakishly large, the other displaced,
but I cannot bear to have them junked
thrice, and let's face it, there's something sexy
about climbing into bed while masquerading
as British counterintelligence and don't we all
know a fondness for things held too long.
We sympathize. Who isn't scratched?
Who among us will never become
grey, square and slightly unbalanced?
With earpieces open, think blue crab.
With earpieces folded, think professor
with arms tucked across the chest.
Visualize the color technician
swirling in ash grey, smoke grey, Berlin blue
and velvet black tints. Feel the intense heat
of plastic decanted into a mold intended
to frame the world, a poetry through which everything
becomes clear and weighs next to nothing.
But as the booklight battery starts to die,
the locust tree of sleep drops blackened pods
and the skinniest volume of poetry

by a woman named Joan begins to weigh
a thousand pounds. The eyelids descend
where no dime-store spectacles can capture
the love-blinded light besmudging leaf
although really there is no Joan and,
strictly speaking, that was no locust tree.

A REFUSAL TO SHARE

Take my organs including kidneys and eyeballs,
memories, closet space, passivity and aggression.
Carry away all possessions in carts like Roman senators,
smash and grab the living room furniture,
rifle the bedroom for hidden deeds and the photo
of a freckled dog. Hook your dogsled
to my home and drag away like in Nova Scotia,
or better yet, why not just move in
and unpack your bags. Borrow my pen.
Fill your plate with gobbledygook, grief,
missing spaces, the painstaking unpraised work,
wretched and commonplace. Eat at my favorite table
at an open air café on Rue St. Germain.
Browse my garage sale of concrete
and sensory detail. Weigh in your hand the knickknack
of clumsy prom moment. Turn your back
on the rack of clothes, jilted again on the driveway
dance floor. Wrinkled gloves, you wear one,
I'll the other. Frayed pants, though we'll have to take turns.
That park bench at Wilder Mansion, slide over.
I will share with you the smell of vinyl pencil case
on the first day of school. Dry socks and wet socks.
Radiator steam. Stuffed peppers, one for each of us,
while we split a bottle of Merlot. The texture of ripe peaches.
My portion of the Pacific Ocean is yours
for the taking, along with a preferred planet,
constellation, all matter and anti-matter. What does it matter
to me? But I will not, cannot, flatly refuse
(putting my foot down here once and for all)
to share her. She of the infinite permutations
of divinity in a dress. Perhaps if I die
I will change my mind (after her decade of mourning
wearing only pitch black). Perhaps instead,
I can interest you in this lime twin popsicle
specifically designed for our purposes.
I'll cut. You choose. Even Stevens. Wallace, that is.

MISPLACED

I set down my keys and they walk,
serrated legs slicing across surfaces
to hide behind an unspeakable volume of Locke
knowing no one would ever lift to browse.
Perhaps they blow like milkweed defying Newton's Law
of Gravity, or disappear in defiance of Lavoisier's Law
of Conservation of Matter. They cavort
with the lost socks under the sofa,
chill with the leftover chicken limone in the frig,
or become edgy as an escaped turtle.
Why they climb into a gym shoe
I'll never figure out. Where do they hope to go?

Eventually I give up, wait for the keys
to fall like an apple from a tree,
knock some sense, some semi-brilliant misplaced idea.
Sometimes they appear after long debauch,
sleep it off on the couch. Return like a bag lunch
uneaten, an opening line, a flashback of a childhood home,
or a dark-eyed woman at a booksellers,
deepening the essential mystery. Why can't they behave
themselves like fruit in a bowl. Still life,
never having started a car with a ripe pear,
leads me to understand their motive for leaving
was pure and that these are exactly
the restless kind of keys I could love.

STRIP MALL

Friday night, after work, I am flying
  down Roosevelt Road so anxious to get home,
never before having felt such love
  for the strip mall, such creative couplings,
optical and pizza, phone and sushi,
  karate, tattoo, mattress, tire,
waxing, cleaners, liquor, donut,
  gaming, dollar, bridal, vaping,
jewelry, mortgage, hearing, pub,
  pet, haircut, wireless, cake.
Who would not welcome Magic Feet?
  Why not Palm Beach Tan?
Bah to all those stuck-up stiffs
  who hold the strip in such disdain!
It's Friday night and I've a date
  with Dar: strip mall date night
to Swarama Express, chiropractor, VCR
  movie repair and rental and, of course,
Sun Nails where I will purchase for her
  a set of nails imprinted with stars and stripes.
She will enjoy Gyroburger, the original
  King Kong, then later leave little red
strip malls down my straightened spine.

ODE TO THE SHELL STATION
A week before Easter, 2020

Thank God, the Cool Ranch Doritos insist
on their necessity. A roll of 6 chocolate glazed mini donuts
    from Little Debbie returns you to your first principles. The Slim Jim,
        named for a tool used for breaking into a locked auto,
is now available with a twin of processed cheese
    to be doubly sure that every coronary artery in every trucker
        traveling route 83 enjoys its own roadblock. You turn

your sympathies to the *Now and Laters,*
hopeful in their bleachers, destined to be jilted again,
    while Sour Patch Kids proliferate. Fortunately, condoms
        are available, including The Magnum for the deluded,
the standard Trojan for the demure, and The Party Pack
  for the completely spazzed-out. Be certain to read
        the fine print on the orange push-up pop

whose makers clearly state there is no actual sherbet,
only imitation sherbet, filling the paper piston,
    in case you were considering legal action. Don't bother
        as they still taste pretty good, as does everything
in this emporium, including the antifreeze which you understand
    has a sweet taste, like Yoohoo, an artificial chocolate drink.
        In coolers, these bottles have been toed up to the starting line

forever. What enviable patience! What optimism!
Even the giant pickles, really just dwarf cucumbers,
    are willing to wade in bags of salt solution and yellow dye
        with the old-fashioned hope of rekindling a memory
of reaching into a barrel up to the shoulder.
    Come celebrate the vulgarity of a jumbo drink cup
        too large to be lifted to a mouth. Tamales

roll on ingenious warming poles, offer greasy seduction.
But wait! You already have a date, as your cellmate
    accepts the offer. She accepts! Recognizing that you are going
        to the Shell Station to top off the Ford Escape,
whether motivated by humanitarian values or the need
  to get out, she cuts a slender silhouette
        in her yoga pants, which have never encountered

Phillip J. Cozzi   35

a yoga mat. She wends her way toward the wine,
holds a bottle at forty-five degrees like the white-coated maître'd
        at Chez Boutin, rotates it on its earthly axis
            and announces the light-yellow fluid has flowed
all the way from New Zealand, boasts a quality
        of any of its kind in Europe. You replace the six-pack
            of Hamms, and head toward Kate who hovers

    behind bullet proof glass. She welcomes your warmth
with a little joke about the end of her shift.
        Missing all but the middle two of her top teeth,
            Kate smiles like the Easter Bunny, glasses askew.
You return to your coronavirus hell
        with Doritos and an elixir of white wine, while she
            has another hour to go. A drug deal

    which occurs between idling autos
in the corner of the parking lot is coming along
        swimmingly. The human mew of the ghost cats
            swells in symphony from behind a dumpster.
You pull away to the crunch of tire on gravel
        in soft rain, the tell-tale pelting of guilt on the hood
            of a car. This cleansing inspires belief,
                like the smell of petrol.

HOW TO USE A CAN OPENER

First, get to know Jan Shrammel,
mother of six grown Shrammels,
and listen carefully to her family traditions,
especially that of the blueberry jello,
covered with blended creme cheese, sour cream,
and chopped pecans. Second, you need
to use your stethoscope to auscultate
her heart, lungs and bowel sounds.
Third, have a personal epiphany
in the parking lot of the Jewel food store,
never having felt such love for the thud-
thud-thudding of car doors. Next,
hunt the kitchen drawers for the can opener,
which waits with peelers and odd-shaped ladles:
a lever with a wheel, simple as birthing tongs.
Finally, bear down with all your weight until
the miracle of the wheel breaks the seal
on the gravid can of Oregon berries gestating
in light syrup. Listen carefully
for the suckling noise, the first breath
in the lungs of newborn blueberries.

HALVES

Hearts or moons or gods as with the half-goat,
half-man, Pan. A cup of sugar. Football games.
The life of my cousin Bella who bounces
from her mother's home to her father's home.
Korea. Confidences. Candy bar, as one kid cuts
and the other chooses. Grilled cheese sandwiches.
Cantaloupe. Siamese twins. But I think
of Alan and Georgie Mayer, my grad school friends,
as a whole, Alan having fallen in love
with Georgie the first time he saw her skin
a rabbit, cutting quickly down the middle,
eviscerating the bunny. Now the undivided guest
at her birthday party, two kids in pointy hats
and grimy highchairs, I learned love also
can be halved by watching Alan slice
the final piece of cake, offer her the bigger half.

PERITEXT

> Peri: 1. a supernatural being in Persian folklore descended from fallen angels and excluded from paradise until penance is accomplished.
>
> 2. a beautiful and graceful girl.
>
> *Webster's Ninth New Collegiate Dictionary*

I like peritext. I like wet socks,
flat tires, cracked ping-pong balls.
I like to sneeze. I like the violence
of the sneeze, at least for that half second,
forgetting all responsibilities and failures.

I like people who write peritext,
words so miniscule they cannot be read,
words from people who rhapsodize in the irony
of written word never intended to be read.
Micrographia is a sign of disease,
but look closer, turn that page
like a microscope slide under a lens
and flagellated protozoan words
scoot across papery pond water.

I like the word peritext, which brings to mind
a graceful impenitent Persian woman.
O the strength and possibilities!
I admire the efficiency of the word text,
2 t's and an ex, and any word
with the letter x, garnering 8 points
on the Scrabble board, so valuable and rare.

Pericardium protects the heart.
Perinatal, perineum, and peripartum
all have to do with birth,
and that beautiful girl will soon nuzzle
in the crook of her mother's arm,
in the reading chair and the safety
of knowing the copyright is protected.
Periwinkle is ground cover, a "European creeper,"

someone that college-bound daughter should avoid.

Everything peripheral perishes like vision
and peritext in books in the junk bin.
So embarrassing. First full priced
then slashed and slashed with magic marker,
until they can't be given away, until
they have to pay someone to cart them away.

Once, while I was backing out
of my parking space, slowly after mass,
I saw the subtlest trace of something
flash by in my peripheral vision, touched
the brakes, and a second later
Patrick Morgan's toddler son emerged
fully into my rearview mirror. For years now,
weekly at mass, still in my peripheral vision,
I have watched that boy, the one
I almost ran over, grow up.
That's the kind of peritext to love.

READING LIANA'S LIPS AT HER GARDEN RECITATION

You could make out only one word, "grandmother,"
her West Indies accent drowned in the chittering,
and had to imagine the wood block kitchen table,
exotic fruit lopped firmly with a quick chop,
halves falling apart as after love,
her evil eye and clothes pinned bedsheets.

You had to trust a mouthed art to summon
the luscious crush of pineapple on tongue,
as her poem held you in its teeth.
Her cheeks: the confident fullness of plums.

Once, you listened in silence while Darlene
signed the gospel according to John
for the Family New Year's Eve Talent Show.
For all you knew, Liana's words were sacred.

For all you knew, she declared love
for the wren in his grey-brown sport coat
who eavesdropped on her reading
knowing for certain that his early flight
did not reflect an opinion on the quality
of her poetry, but rather inspiration.

Her words spread like seed by birds
which ate the fruit, and what you loved most
about the poem was how her lips
retracted tightly against the teeth
every time she mouthed the "ee" sound,

like the silence of a child sinking
into a grandmother's broad Caribbean lap.

ON THE CRITICISM MARY NEEDS A NEW WORD FOR "HUM"

The word "hum" is numb
like thumb and dumb and begs
to be booted, scooted, rooted,
escorted down the plank, a skank,
picked like nit, flicked with finger,
pulled like a fallen hair
from sweater. You can do better.
No hum-drum, ho-hum humming.
We need words. Real words
not turds, dodo birds, flat tires,
fat squires. We don't care
what mother thrums at the kitchen sink,
your father's music while he shaves.
We think the weakling verb behaves
a chore, a boar in any war. No spit,
no fist, no twisted vowel, no disembowel.
We want martyr, spicy tarter,
word that tries a little harder.
We want dazzle, frazzle,
bite through muzzle, shoot from nozzle,
forge the mysteries, then puzzle.
So we scalpel, shackle, wail, waltz
the wimpling off to jail,
where prison gangs with fangs call dibs
to shove a shiv beneath its ribs.

 Phillip J. Cozzi

EULOGY

Adverb was a good word.
Everyone loved him, wonderful spouse
to his beloved verb. Father to six.
On Saturdays, he cut his lawn. Sundays,
he slept. Accepted work without complaint.
Never said a cross word. Humble
were his beginnings: adopted by Dickens,
became parlor favorite to Hawthorne,
but never one of the cool kids, never invited
to the movable feast, fell victim to shunning
by post-moderns and now is dead as Dickens.
Sure, at the end of novels, he smiled strangely
or left abruptly, but when he carried you
to bed, lifting without waking, he did so
                                    tenderly.

After the wake, the adjectives
piled into their clown car,
decided to skip the luncheon.
It didn't take long before the word *petty*
cracked a joke and they all cackled
                                    maniacally.

LATE-NIGHT CHECK-IN AT THE TRILLIUM MOTEL

You hate wildflowers for always flaunting
impossible names, always pimping
on life cycle, always preaching
rich purple or fiery red sermons:
"Why are you wasting your life?"
or "Communicating with nature."
You can take a maximum of 15 minutes
before hunting the hotel bar
for a play-off game and nature's stunning beauty
in full bloom. Makes you want
to kick that scientist in the balls
for categorizing, using Latin names,
the way you should respond the way he responds
to fungus and moist soil. Let's face it:
it's all about sex and trickery –
woodland floors and hotel bars.
They remind you of a girl you dated
in school, who hung your hand-picked bouquet
upside down on her bedroom wall
knowing it dries better that way
and now, God damn it,
you can't remember her name either.
Of course, wildflowers are lovely but
that's not the point. The point is
they make you feel like an insect,
late-night check-in at the trillium motel,
just before the flower closes for the day,
unclear if you are trapped
or have decided to spend the night
wrapped in the petal's embrace.

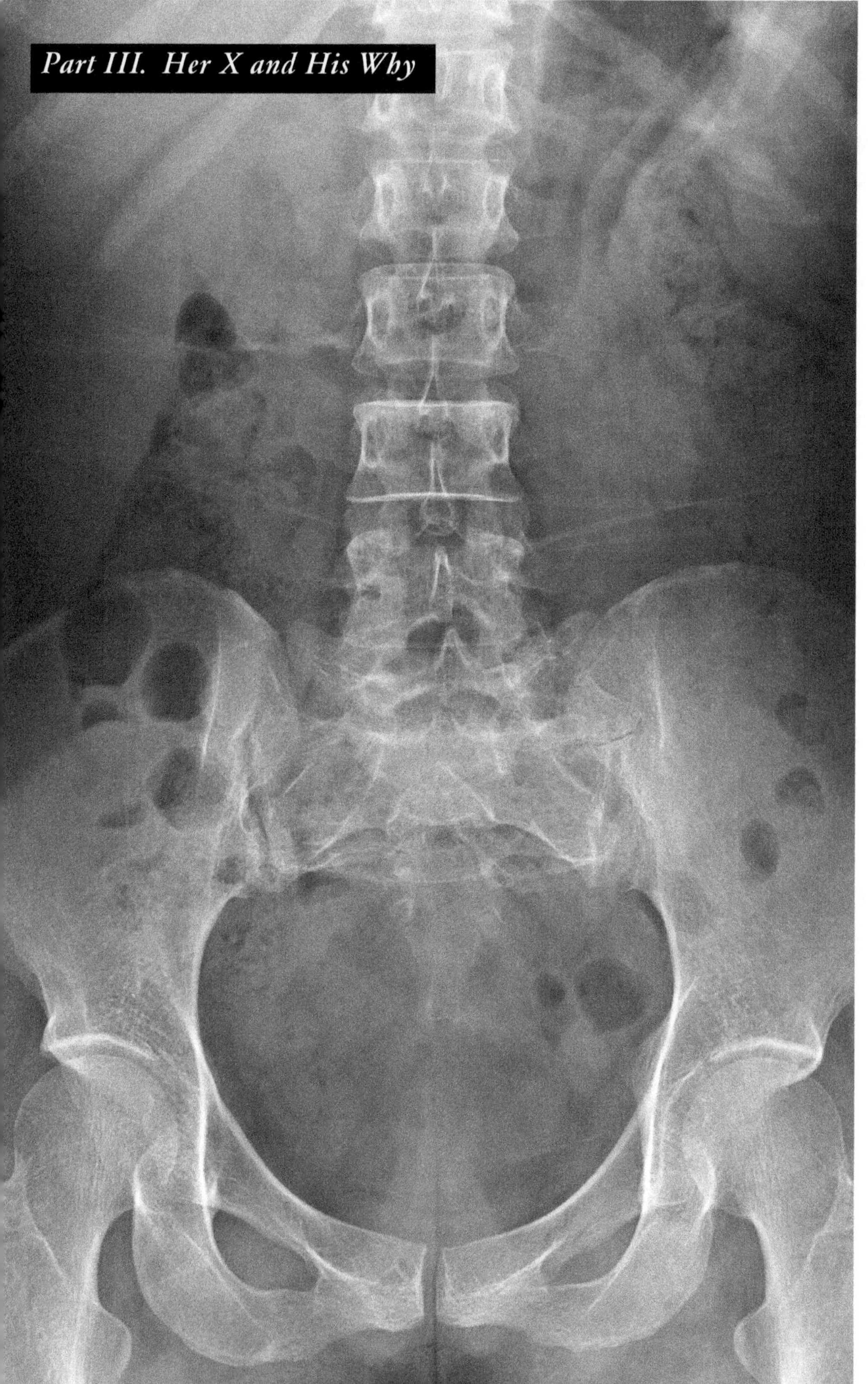

Part III. Her X and His Why

PINK OWL

I read the flashcard "baseb,b,b,ball."
The woman in glasses frowned until time ran out
then my mother and I walked to the Rexall
at the bus stop. I chose a Pink Owl
Bubble Gum cigar. That moment, my mother
all to myself, holds power over me today,
fluent fingers entwined with the strength
of silence, no need for speech, far away
from the pill bottles of candy, sandbag ashtrays
brimming with the ashes of angers,
the clever, loud voices. I knew exactly
why I stuttered but could not sssssssay.

I TOLD MY MOTHER SHE WAS GOING TO DIE

A celebration of subtlety, my mother's life
was a hint unrecognized, a parting
of the lips, modest as weekday meals,
the longings of laundry and a kettle of quietude,
quiet not silent, a simmering one cannot hear
unless listening carefully. She always wore
her hair in the style of Veronica Lake,

a simple barrette holding the part in blonde
framing of the face, classic without trying,
graduated from Freeman Secretarial School
in an era of shoe polish and scraping skies,
before retiring at 25, with the first of 8.
I was the sixth, the physician, and the first

of 3 cancers announced itself with blood
from the nipple. The melanoma she mistook
for a burn from her iron, curling too close
to her ear. Finally, pancreatic cancer knocked
as an ingénue at the producer's door.

We chose the living room to discuss death,
a place previously reserved for prom dates
and keeping malignant relatives at bay.
"This can be cured?" she asked of one

blind to the light who refused
to shine. Her pulse: the tapping
at a typewriter's heart. She was diagnosed

demure, nuanced all that slams
and veers with the hook

and hush of acceptance.

PERISCOPE

My mother bought Cap'n Crunch
as she knew I wanted the periscope,
made from cereal box, cut along dashed lines,
folded, fitted with tin foil, an eyepiece,
and, Wham! Junior sleuth,
able to see around corners, ready
to foil counterfeiters and smugglers.
They never worked but I knew
all about periscopes from 1960's submarine shows,
Richard Basehart and the declaration "Up, periscope!"
just before the Russian torpedo slammed
the hull. Alarms sounded. The camera shook
while sailors scrambled claustrophobic gangways
so that all of America would not bear witness
to the most awful death imaginable.
We sailed into the 21st century
before pancreatic cancer torpedoed
our South Oak Park brick bungalow.
For the next 11 months, 8 kids
scuttled hallways. And God,
in His mercy infinite, whispered wordlessly
that I should climb into bed with her,
on the night before she died,
just like we always did,
sometimes all 8 of us at once,
like King Oscar sardines submerged
in salt water. Until she fell asleep,
I hugged her, able at last to see
around corners and the next bad guy coming.

BIRTHDAY CAKE for WARNICE

My father chugged his chicken-pocked Chrysler,
this rust spotted leper, through the neighborhood
as if giving the finger to everyone,
with myself complicit in the front seat,
sloshing toward Entenmann's factory outlet
which looked deceased a half century ago.
Broken cookies, bungled pies, jilted cakes pined
in this orphanage for passed up pastry
sold for pennies. It was my birthday,
December 17, 1966 and I pitied
the lumps of dough, the forlorn walnut
coffee cakes stale at birth, but my father
loved this place. Such bargains!
We landed a beaute: white sheet cake
with purple lettering which mortified
my mother. My sibs were glutted with laughter
as my father scraped off the birthday wishes
for Warnice with a butter knife. Now, 50
years later, I want to find you, Warnice,
like a biological mother or my twin separated
at birth. Might be sweet to know you,
hold you squarely by the shoulders, give thanks
for sharing, long-late birthday wishes
and this slice of your own life vicariously lived.

Phillip J. Cozzi   49

THE OLD SWITCHEROO

My father is made of mucilage,
backscratcher, shoehorn, cigar box,
paper clip, rubber band, styptic pencil,
mechanical pencil, the Hair-Wiz, toothpick,
a fat wad of singles bound with a rubber band,
gooseneck desk lamp, shoebox Easter basket,
silver penny, wide tie, sport coat,
ledger paper, pipe cleaner, postage stamp,
a dusty construction-paper miniature burro.
    When he lumbered up the basement stairs,
        struggling like an air conditioner in 100° heat,
            he never failed to act surprised when I leapt
                from my hiding place. He is now kept,
and so frail I could pull the old switcheroo

and carry him on *my* shoulders
'round the three front rooms.

 Phillip J. Cozzi

BAD TOUPEE

I pray before you, blank faced Styrofoam bust
wearing my father's hairpiece, ageless on his dresser.
My sister Peggy drew that pencil-thin moustache
below your molded, generic nose.
Pretending not to notice the lie
for fifty years was easy as I respected
both your willingness to be absurd
and endurance of illusion.
What bald Italian man is reborn blonde
at 85? Any Roman centurion would
envy the artwork on your head,
which says in textured language of hair,
"Hey beautiful" and "Looking good there,"
and even as his muscles evanesced,
face thinned, sport coat hung
as if on skeleton, and the rug rumpled
when two-way tape no longer gripped
greasy scalp, you reminded each morning
"You are powerful and deserving,
present and have never been more
authentically yourself." Praise be
to this sainted icon of manhood!

Phillip J. Cozzi 51

CHASING OLIVES

A combined 188 years old, my father's hands
don't work. He holds his fork too close
to the end, like a dart, and chases
an olive around his plate as it traverses
an oil slick shaped like South America.
Playful and stubborn, the stone and meat
will not relent. When I make suggestion,
his sideways glance informs me
both "Stay out of this,"and "I'm having
too much fun." Two opponents, each
thick-skinned, one on one ancient warriors
in a mini porcelain coliseum
with survival at stake. I read of a man
who traveled to every country on the planet
for *The Happiness of Pursuit*. This
my father found on a Wednesday night
at Al's Restaurant on Cermak Road.

 Phillip J. Cozzi

MODERN POETRY

"What is this crap?"
my father blurts out and I tell him,
for the third time, "This is spaghetti,"
which, of course, does not look like spaghetti
as it is pureed. It does not taste or feel
like spaghetti. It does smell faintly of spaghetti
but not enough to trigger a memory
of his mother, Rafaela, square-framed, always
in a simple print dress, always salted water
boiling, always the taste of poise amid chaos.
Or his weighty father explaining the gravity
of the proper technique of using the spoon
in rolling the noodles on the fork and the delight
in his son's new-found skill. At one time, my father
loved the words "al dente," "bolognaise." Today,
even the crisp voice of the noodle is replaced
with the unintelligible growl of the blender,
the lines disappearing into mush. I encourage,
"Give it a chance, dad." "One more spoonful."
and "This is good for you." Between spoonfuls,
I read him poetry, as he has always loved
poetry. I lift my modern poetry magazine
into focus and spoon out the words.

ORACLE

My father walks on five legs.
Stop right there. How could Homer
describe the person yet no such word
existed until the Middle Ages? Do you mean
to tell me the deities spoke through men
and women for over a thousand years
and those enchanted remained unnamed
but clearly existed? My brother, Bob,
for example, prophesied the fall,
the spiral fracture, the "I got bad news"
phone call, the rodding and recovery.
Using a walker, hopping on one leg,
my 94 year old father, minus the toupee,
created a new word today: *daylightwhale.*
Nearly insane, from stopping him
for the 110th time from pulling out his IV,
I puzzled at this oracle. What
mischievous god, both snapped his tibia
and bewitched his tongue, fluent
in both gibberish and genius, and cast
my mind on the heaving seas of ancient
Leviathans, horrific and magnificent,
breaching so high in the air, their
liquid frames filled with light?

FLIRT

My father was a terminal flirt
even deep into his eighties and nineties.
He liked women. I saw this early.
How he paid extra attention
to young, mini-skirted neighbor wives.
I saw this in his middle age,
with clients and his friend's wives.
A decade after my mother passed,
we did a father/son weekend,
just the boys at Pheasant Run.
At 89, he sported a blonde toupee
and a wide tie in a Windsor knot.
A handsome young couple, hand in hand,
jumbled into the elevator with us.
My father sized her up shamelessly,
joked, "You're not with him, are you?"
She was hooked, bought mojitos poolside,
chased him down at The Look Out Bar and,
when she tried to join us for brunch,
he leaned over in his wheelchair
and whispered, "Get me outta here."
Six days before his 96th birthday,
as he became more and more cantankerous,
I could not calm him down.
My wife took his head in her hands,
placed her face 6 inches from his
and smiled fetchingly, "It's alright, Sweetheart."
In an instant, he relaxed, laid back
                              and died.

X

After my Dad died I discovered the letter "x" raising little arms in praise for his easy
  passing
and this letter arrived as a gift an inheritance so to speak which I presume my father
  left
with his sly sense of humor and eyes smiling to see irony which no one else could
  see

After my Dad died the obligatory day came to sift through his most painfully
  personal
items Valentine's Day cards from my mother report cards drawings from children
  diapers
not for children photo of school class his birth certificate with a different first
  name

After my Dad died I discovered the letter "x" in the form of an encyclopedia a
  slender
volume number 24 for the 24th letter of the alphabet which he had reshelved
  upside down
knowing I would be drawn to this reversal this un-expectation I knew he would
  enjoy

and whether he did this knowingly or not I would like to think he left this gift this
  wealth
because haven't we all experienced such post-humous ascensions among those we
  loved
deified immortalized given false attributes and dipped by the heel into sticky
  sentiment

by the musty set of The American Peoples Encyclopedia from which his 8 children
  paraphrased aka plagiarized
their middle school book reports copyright 1966 including my legendary
  "Jet Engines"
replete with plasticene protective cover but now the entire set grins like Alfred E.
  Newman

insipid teethy but missing one tooth as on this day I thumbed the pages of the
  Xingu
River entry which courses through Brazil which has a "z" but sadly alas no
  x
which garners 8 points on the scrabble board and also serves as Roman numeral
  X

originating from the Latin coin denarius meaning "ten asses" perhaps plundered by
  Persian King Xerxes I,
who was lucky enough to have 2 "x"s in his first name but unlucky enough to be
  murdered
by the captain of his guards but lucky again to be succeeded by his son
  Antexerxes

also doubly blessed with "x"s and why I wanted to name my second son
  Xavier
although my conniving wife who worked at St Xavier's College had drawn me a
  snifter
of cognac I who don't even drink or know what a snifter is conceded to
  name

my son after her dead mother Josephine bringing to mind Xantippe wife of the
  Greek
philosopher Socrates who was notorious for her quarrelsome temper and xylene
  a solvent
and not a woman's name Xenophobia Xenophanes Xenocrates (Plato's student)
  Xanthomatosis

(medical speak for high cholesterol) the XYZ affair Xylophone and the everlasting
  Xanthos
one of two immortal horses struck dumb by the Furies for spilling the beans to
  Achilles
that guess what he was not immortal that one day having been dipped like an
  ice cream

cone into chocolatey candy topping he too would melt all slobbery and
  human
as his xrays in the ER graphically demonstrated a poison arrow embedded in his
  heel
a sign post to the door through which each hero must
  exit.

After my Dad died I removed the orange DNR form taped to the side of his
  refrigerator
on which he had scratched a tremulous wholly indecipherable signature at the
  X
so that paramedics would not assault his chest in the masterful exercise of their
  calling

but allow the passing of an ex-living ex-human ex-being who would have
  delighted
in the tragic irony of dying in which the full significance of a life is clear to everyone
  but
the dying and that I reshelved the volume "X" upside down but an "x" is the same if
  inverted

and the extraordinary irony that he chose the name Paul when he could have chosen
  Xerxes X
and who but me remains to apologize for this curiosity having inherited my mother's
  X and his why

IN PRAISE OF MY PARENTS

My mother and father are not artists,
never dwell on love or loss, have none
of the natural elegance of the effete.
My mother does not throw roses out
an open window. My father never arrives
soaking wet at her slum, driven through
heavy rain. They do not picnic
at the Luxembourg Gardens. She does not pose
nude in his studio, charmingly direct
but reticent, nor does she haunt his memory.
He does not appear in her memoir,
tightening scarf about throat. My parents
do not conceal themes, intentionally confuse.
They do not unveil souls, spark divine,
cut though dreams, nor spill the visceral grind.
They do not glow, char, prowl, twist,
divulge, nor gutter like candle.
They do not desolate, harsh, supple.

My mother made superb meatballs.
My father whistled in endless strata,
arabesques in bluish and rosy tones. But
now they are everywhere.
My mother and father are not artists.
They are not tortured, never were.
They are, however, happy, this
tragic consequence of lives together.

LAYING TRACKS
For Joseph Masterson, my grandfather

Dear Joseph, you don't know me
but uncertainty interests me
like the hole in every immigrant stomach,
the line between myth and remembrance,
the reason we finish stale Blatz beer,
the circumstances of your death
in the railyard, 90 years ago,
your widow's unknowing what to do,
your child's questioning, why I picture
a jaunty man down on his haunches
petting a dog, why I write
to my mother's father with the hope
this missive will offer reassurance
everything turned out OK, why a man
laying tracks is alive one second, dead
forever, why in our toil we turn
our backs on the deafening approach
of uncertainty, and why there is beauty
in dropping your namesake at Union Station
on his way back to school by train.

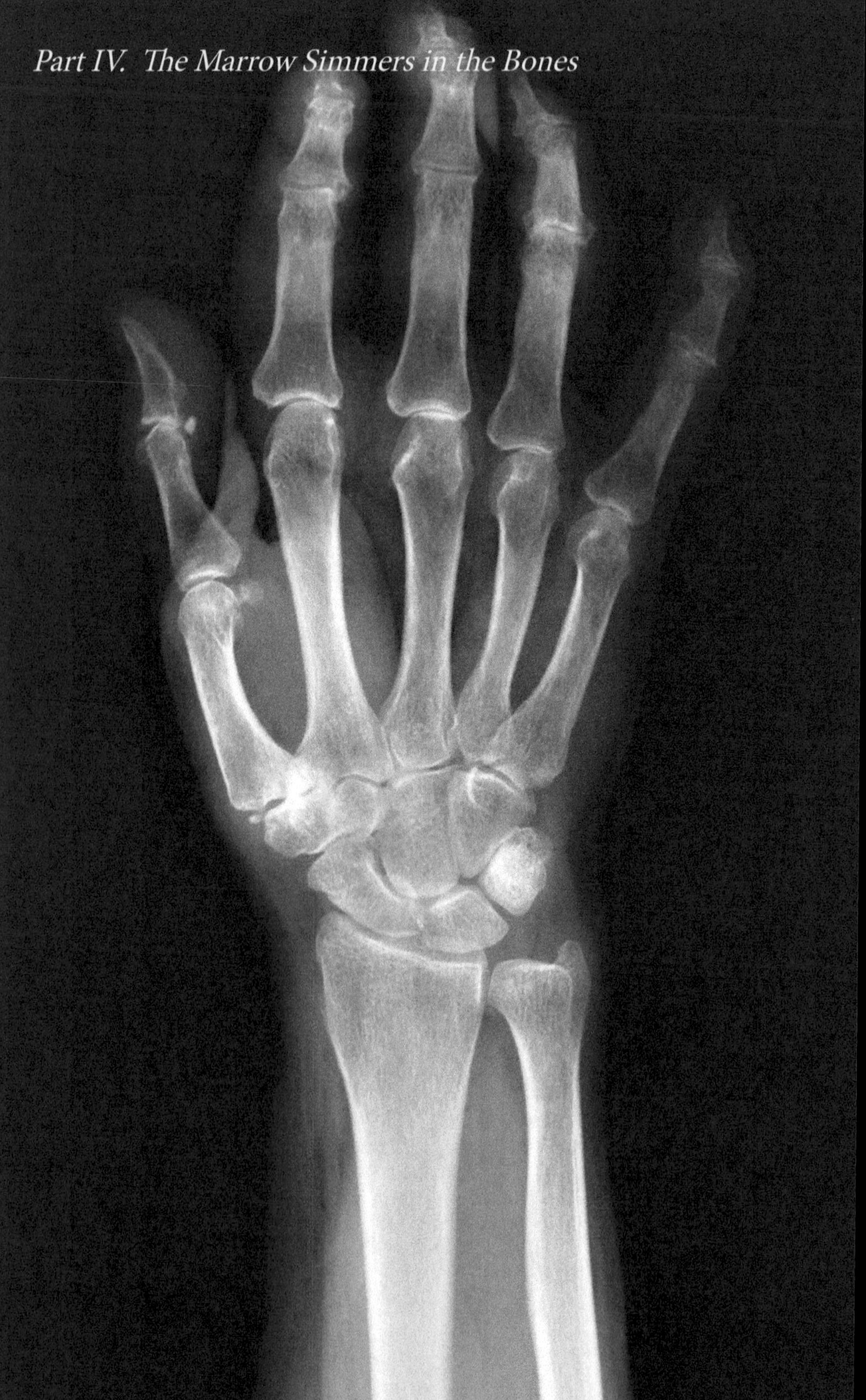
Part IV. The Marrow Simmers in the Bones

FELLOWS

For Cons

It's never easy knowing what to choose,
especially in a light rain. Should you lose
a stroke by chipping to the fairway? Should you drive
on through the trees? We'll both arrive
eventually, beginners always, though we've played
from Spring to Fall with rented clubs.
Your shameless Frosty the Snowman dance
has lost effect. It's almost chance,
your choosing in the woods, but be prepared
to duck in case your choosing fires back
against the trees to rattle like a pinball
on its bumpers. Our discussion by the pond
ripples with the woman from Vermont you call
each night. I watch you fall in love
with my Chicago skyline. Mallards play,
procrastinate, as we go back and forth:
practice or research, money or mankind,
kids or career. In refuge from
the ritualistic beating it endures,
we find your Spaulding 2, an egg
within a nest of pale blue butterwort
beside a row of elderbush, the seeds of which
are spread with birds that eat their fruit.
By muffling rain, the woodland hooch
allows the birdfoot violet voice:
you will not linger long with me
among the oak, azalea, wisteria and nameless
other underbrush. Monseuir Frostaceous,
in his taunting, will achieve. You know
I favor chipping from the woods
and getting safely into play, for happiness
is dog-legged to the left. Or right. Your guess
is as good as mine. I can see you now,
the itinerant pro, playing the great courses
of Bethesda, Boston, over wide-raked traps
with every slash, every unlock of the wrists,

hoping for daylight and big hitting down
narrow and fast-running fairways.

DOCTOR THOMMES AND DOCTOR WOODS

These men of biology are gone.
No more racing to the hatchery
on day thirteen and a half
of incubation. They knitted
experiments with test tubes,
drilled windows in chicken eggs
with a dentist's drill,
dissected and transplanted
each other's thoughts,
wrote and re-wrote,
typed and stapled their studies.
They harvested, fixed, embedded with wax,
sectioned, stained and studied
the glands of unborn birds.

I remember how they kicked me
out of their lab. Then took me back.
They made me laugh with frequent
irrelevant references to the papal monkeys.

Now, at the end of the day,
after my last patient has left,
I turn off the light in the clinic—
in that moment in the dark
they are with me,
lab coats stained,
hands raw from washing glassware,
and the soft smoke of chicken shell fills my nostrils.

ON VIEWING *THE ANATOMY LESSON*

When I see the men with wigs,
pallid faces, slender hands and noses
gaze with only intellect upon the dead,

their learning tool, their hands-on lab,
some look blandly into the chest
where others probe with long instruments

gaining best exposure for the back
row of the auditorium and retract
the meat of the mediastinum,

Puritans robed for turkey dinner,
one dead patient ripe for stuffing,
when I see their keen indifference

I see my own face among them,
cutting nose and guilty eyes,
expressionless.

Please God lift my painted hand
to wipe the long-dried blood from his side
and drape my sterile apron across his face.

 Phillip J. Cozzi

ODE

Simplicity's champion,
penlight's companion,
fruit of the Earth
and tool of the trade
between finger and thumb,
you have not succumbed.

Forthright and elegant
gagger of children,
mover of tongues
and tickler of tonsils,
you bullyboy change
and aging technology.

Today, I schedule scans,
write self-defensive notes,
but you, inflexible friend,
godlike in your constancy,
metaphor for my hero,
insignia of an era,
sentinel standing on end
in a covered glass jar
by the clinic room door,
symbolize our work:
twin to a popsicle stick,
wooden martyr that we
who look inward see.

A CARDIAC SILHOUETTE SEEN ON CHEST X-RAY

Birdhouse squash or buffalo head.
A half-deflated basketball,
A fist, gourd, a sack of seed
Out all night in the rain.

A triangle with corners trimmed,
The sack a Santa carriers,
A boy with both knees pulled
Tight up under his chin.

A plum, a pear or mango fruit,
An amber drop, misshapen,
A saddle purse or betel nut,
Walnut in its shell.

A chocolate-covered cherry treat,
The partly open cotton boll,
Gum drop, teardrop, apricot,
Grapes dangled in bunches.

A drawstring purse, fig or face,
The outline of a fishhook,
The summer haystacks by Monet,
Embryo, ellipse.

An uncut gem, an eyeball, egg,
Potbelly stove on legs,
A glob of dough, a dodo bird.
Hard cheese hung at market.

A racket head, a radish root,
A horse's hoof unshod,
A knob, a jug or one wood club,
Water balloon midair.

 Phillip J. Cozzi

A garlic clove, a gyroscope,
Marzipan or bassinet
Or listen with your stethoscope:
Bell or bagpipe, castanets.

YOUR LOWER EXTREMITIES

The marrow simmers in the bones.
The bones are wrapped in muscled skin
And fibers strap the knee to join
Your thigh to calf and lower limb.
The vessels lie beneath the points
Of nerve and fat and fascial sheath
Which course beyond the ankle joints
To move, mechanically, the feet.
Yet when I see your figure move
From room to room or rise from chair
My learned knowledge only leaves
The muscled beauty walking there.
Although attractive science begs
I can't deny I love your legs.

CLINIC CHART

Log of your snifflings,
manilla memoir of athletic misadventure,
ship's journal of travel immunizations,
English novel in which our hapless protagonist, Yourself,
triumphs over the villainy of allergic rhinitis.

The plastic tabs of life stick out,
conveniently, so as to divide you
into drug lists, labs, x-rays,
the lofty literature of consultants,
and, most optimistically, the progress notes,
that periodical of a vagabond physique,
minutes to a lifelong meeting.

Accounts from hemorrhoids to heart disease
are published in this confidential press.
No scandal sheet or junk tabloid,
it reads like war correspondence,
you covering the grenade with your helmet,
I tapping code over wires.

Chronicle of your constitution.
The chapter on cholecystitis,
the fiction of your heart's flutterings,
the subplot of dyspepsia,
the suspense of "hot eyeballs,"
the epiphany of Lyme disease phobia,
the denouement of reactive depression.

Minor characters accompany you
or wait demurely in my lobby,
thumbing the worthless teen gazettes,
while the real literature,
that perfect art reflecting life,
those immodest scribblings,
address the unsolved mysteries:

Phillip J. Cozzi   **69**

your insomnia and
that metal taste in your mouth.

So here I am again today,
your steadfast scrivener,
your biased biographer,
pen in hand and a white cloud
dallying in the window at my back,
ready for another entry,
the latest peregrinations of my hero.

 Phillip J. Cozzi

STRANGER'S HEART

My brother Larry is alive but his counterpart
is not.
        I keep remembering
the trauma dock doors, bright afternoon

light pouring through
        beckoning, almost saying:

run in cut-offs through a sprinkler,
strip to the waist and shoot hoops,
comb the alleys on stingray bikes.

And, thinking back, I realize the sirens,
the same we had always heard, sounded somehow
hollow, somehow different.
        By two, the pace of the shift
was picking up; a call came:
injuries, guard rail, estimated time of arrival.

When the stretcher brushed past me,
garish red light flashed on cheek and temple:

I swear I saw my brother's face

and the brutality of metal, ribs flailing, lung and heart
exposed. We had seen wrecks almost as brutal; we
all had been brushed by
        stretchers moving
past, disasters unexplained. Only moments later
did I know

Larry was alive and elsewhere. Elsewhere.

Then love for my brother welled up inside me.
I who have never hugged my brother,

never kissed him,
          never given speech
to that love, and I realized this

while massaging a stranger's heart.

SONNET FOR SHIRLEY

Drizzling rain at 4 PM. It's sad to know
you're lying to my face. Amid the stink
of alcohol, I fill your forms, although
you're not as sick as you would make me think.
Your name is Shirley Jones, but you are not
the girl from Carousel. The common cold
and disability is yours: you thought
your acting talents suited the role.
But Shirley, you should know that I have lied
to you for I am powerless to treat
the underlying illnesses which lead
so many to this sad deceit, and that,
despite my arrogance, I have no cure
while poverty is drizzling everywhere.

HAZEL ESCAPES ON A ROPE MADE OF BEDSHEETS

Hazel, from her death bed, reached up, grabbed me
by the lapel, pulled me six inches from her face
to read the Dr's name on my white lab coat,
made the observation that her name has only one "z,"
while my name has two. But it was the way
she said it, the wry sense, the sly timing
and comic weight to her mugged expression,
holding me until I registered the absurdity,
her feigned importance to the discovery
of having been slighted at birth. Family
wanted hospice, then recanted, then hospice
again. And who would not equivocate while
the cobalt glint in her iris invoked
zygote to zephyr? She released me to ponder
a name beginning with the exclamation "Ha"
or half a laugh, grounded to the lightning
angled "z," ending with "el" as in El Greco
or that crowded train car in which we all sit
in mute vigil, hoping to get home soon.
But not so fast! The next AM, Hazel arrived,
chipper, leaned into pureed French Toast,
in this story which refused conclusion.
Had she dreamed that night of shimmying down
a rope made of bedsheets, making off
with her massive broken heart, bulging
like ripe fruit or an old ladies' purse?
Did the wild rhododendrons applaud?
Did flaxflower bend with laughter at the bare
backside of a comedienne in a hospital gown
slipping past spotlights to the outstretched arms
of an audience of silver maples?

 Phillip J. Cozzi

BEATING COVID

The nasty little fucker said
I like to kill Hispanics. Reynaldo lifted
his head from the pillow
to the most subtle degree.
We were in the basement
of Memorial Hospital
in a makeshift ICU.
81 COVID patients
in a 39-bed unit. After
I'm done with you,
I'll get your wife. But
I don't have a wife,
Reynaldo said. Then
I'll kill your mother.
Then I could see
a determination on Reynaldo's face
as if his limp body
were to spring fast
from the sick bed
and throw a frenzy
of punches, bare-knuckled,
again and again,
as the spiteful prick stumbled
backward like the meanest bastard
foreman in a fight
on the docks. Then Reynaldo's head
very very slowly eased
back into his pillow.
He looked up at me
like a fighter on his stool
looking at the cut man.
His face softened and,
with a voice gravelly
and strangely quiet
from having survived intubation
for 23 days, he said, Hey doc
how are you holding up?

FIRST CLINIC VISIT WITH MR. SHRAMMEL

The last time I saw him,
encephalopath, addict to ethanol,
his soft accent had been replaced
by a dirge of ventilator valves
opening and closing in chorus.
His hair was a greasy mat
and his sheepish, guilty, half-hidden grin
had fallen open, a mouth incapable
of subtlety. Even the sweet
stink of his breath
was gone.

But the first time I saw Mr. Shrammel
when sunlight poured into the clinic
like a draught of beer
and shone on that likable grin
and the hair he claimed to comb
with Danish butter, straight back,
when his breath spoke more of perfume
than poison, I thought
I am so lucky
to be in medicine.

 Phillip J. Cozzi

POPSICLE

Remember running in cutoffs on hot hot summer afternoons
directly across neighbor's lawns, through sprinklers, across curbs,
toward the jingling bells and the man in white hustling
treats from the side of a truck. We were stunned into silence
by the vast array of choices. Wahoo bars, only five cents.
Who could afford a toasted almond bar? Nothing compared
to a sloppy melting lime or banana twin Popsicle.
Twin Popsicles, best separated on the edge of a table
by a quick hit with the ball of the hand, were twice as good.
Remember sucking the end so hard that all the juice ran up
and out, leaving only a white skeleton of a Popsicle.
We each negotiated the final nubbin of frozen ice
on stick in individual ways. So it didn't surprise me,
thirty years later, to learn that Mr. Bowers requested,
five minutes before support was withdrawn, a Popsicle,
as if reveling in the choices remaining for him
and all the dying. He ran back through time
to the squish of feet on watered grass,
the luscious crush of Popsicle on tongue.

Phillip J. Cozzi 77

CONCERNING EMMA

I want to speak with you concerning Emma.
Pupils fixed, vent-dependent, she lives
as a swollen eggplant on its stem.
I understand you gave her many joys,
sixty years of prior health,
a strong voice and will, and I think you
must be very proud of her who
independently returned respect to you.
I know you are very busy and
I do not want to hold you further,
but now that I am entrusted
with her care I need your help
for though I met her only late
I must tend the leaf as best I can
and, anticipating other seasons, turn the soil.

 Phillip J. Cozzi

BURNING OUT

First you lose respect for the limbs,
then abdomen, then lungs and heart,
and ultimately, you're happily hacking at brain
in search of your corpse's pituitary stalk.

Years later, you suddenly realize that
your breast exams are faster than your speech.
Position sense, vibration, hot and cold,
the cranial nerves have gone the way of the fundus:
a willing suspension of recognition.

Soon your exam consists of senseless pokes
at the pannus of the belly and knee jerks,
which will be the next to go. Words
like "fremitus" and "pectoriloquy" float
like clouds on the surface of a river
headed out to join the differential
of pheochromocytoma and the faces
of forgotten patients.

VOICES OF THE ICU

Grab me with one hand and throw me
across your doorway, let my hooks rattle.
Let my neat hem hide the suffering
like a shared blindfold to all who pass,
stitched so that pain may be private.
Let my creaseless self transform from sheet
to new love, guardian of your solitude,
keeper of most vulnerable vulnerability,
woven wall of moralistic thread,
thou shall not share thy body with the world.

I am fabled, sharp and hollow,
disposable, efficient, evil,
wanting so to be inside you,
wanting so to give you life.
Once our famous interlude:
you were bruised and I forgotten.
Look away. My life is over,
heaped within a common grave.

Confusion is a piece of glass
dividing space. Why bisect
arbitrarily the clarity of a morning
born whole and wanting to be one?
I cut the air like one-armed scissors,
no more concerned than a child clipping comics.
I am the blind eye through which you see.

I am a lover of wrists and bedrails, giver of slack
and restraint and if mornings are shackled
in leather weeds and evenings suffer
the limitations of light in dusk,
you too will suffer my tease of slack.

Town crier to which nobody responds,
I have seen too many wolves in dreams:
everywhere I look, a heart stops,

 Phillip J. Cozzi

a breath stalls. Good news,
even good news, is spoken so disturbingly
that even the mother could not love
the voice of this most colicky child.

I will track through your head
travel to your bowels, provide suction
or sustenance. It hurts that you of all
should hate me most taped to your nostril.
I want so much for you and that you
might find within your stiffened heart
the kindness to recognize my utility.

If your mother is a stainless steel box,
virgin eyes blank as gauges,
passion parceled as air and blown
from her lips into your own,
then you will be cradled in hollow arms
or buckled in this runway buggy
until you learn to toddle again,
liberated from my terrible breast.

Your father's love has two upright beams
and a transom. Though my frame is huge,
there is absolute emptiness inside
unless you fill my threshold. I offer
no more certainty on either side,
But my love is to release you to risk
and my sadness and joy is to lift your veil,
kiss you and give you away
standing before the altar with the world.

Phillip J. Cozzi 81

APPLE CORE LESION

As brothers, we fought in the crab apple wars
using garbage can lids for our shields.
When beaned upon the head, we could only pretend
that it didn't hurt as badly as it did.
We'd take a few bites of the apple first
then throw it back as hard as we could.

But this time was different: forty years later,
one apple sailed through the slats of the fence
which for years has encircled our home.
Now cancer remains on our dining room
table like unwanted fruit in a bowl.

I wish we could fight in the crab apple wars
again and, knowing what we know, might bring
a different strategy into the trees
that bear our symbols of life and death.

LOVE POEM OF THE RURAL DOC

Because he loved his work, he suffered.
Loved to suffer and suffered to love
and suffered to know the work of love
as he had suffered the love of work
until finally he assumed their suffering,
heel driven against the blade, he shoveled
great spoonfuls into his pickup truck
until it sagged beneath the weight
spilling into every corner of the bed.
He drove the tired fields at the edge
of town. It was dusk. The sweep
of wind was the only music.
Whorled line of square hands loved
the labor of the shovel handle as
he unloaded what he could, then with
the bed-door open, sped through the fields
leaving a cloud like duster plane
and as the suffering settled, he kept driving,
one hand on the wheel, one out the window,
chill filtering between his fingers, but
it didn't matter. Nothing mattered because
he was exhausted and he was in love.

***

Vroom. Vroom. Does he see a mountain
of tomatoes? Two helium balloons surprise him
as he opens the trunk. The pictorial encyclopedia
of Civil War equipment, written by a dentist,
plays in the forefront, while Chris drags
a small felled tree to the garbage in the background.
Chris is 3 years old. Who will put the fruit away?
He thanks goodness the other kids are sleeping
or the love of his life would never understand
pretend reading in speech-language-impaired children.
The guilt of changing shoes before leaving for the E.R.

Phillip J. Cozzi   83

***

To conclude the evening hours, he performs
a complete physical on Mrs. Ruth Hartigan
then closes up, walks home. Along the way,
a sense of belonging circulates the dirt-veined town.
Visitors can palpate this. Basketballs percuss
gravel driveways. Four-wheeled bicycles graze
the lawns, fat purple handgrips antler their frames.
Dry weeds digest the edge of every home,
ossified in place. The neighbor's words lick
with canine sensitivity, while moths soften
the lamplights, perfected in the sky.
He lives here. He has no choice.
This town grips him like ivy.
Ambivalence, anguish, couplings, revenge,
to which he is privy, glue the pieces, artwork
shown at the children's farm district fair.
It is not difficult to love this work:
crepe and Elmer's, lives in fingerpaint.
Mrs. Hartigan's red handprint is
the blossom on his construction paper tulip
and the moon floats in their tea cups.
O yes, loving them all equally, the moon.

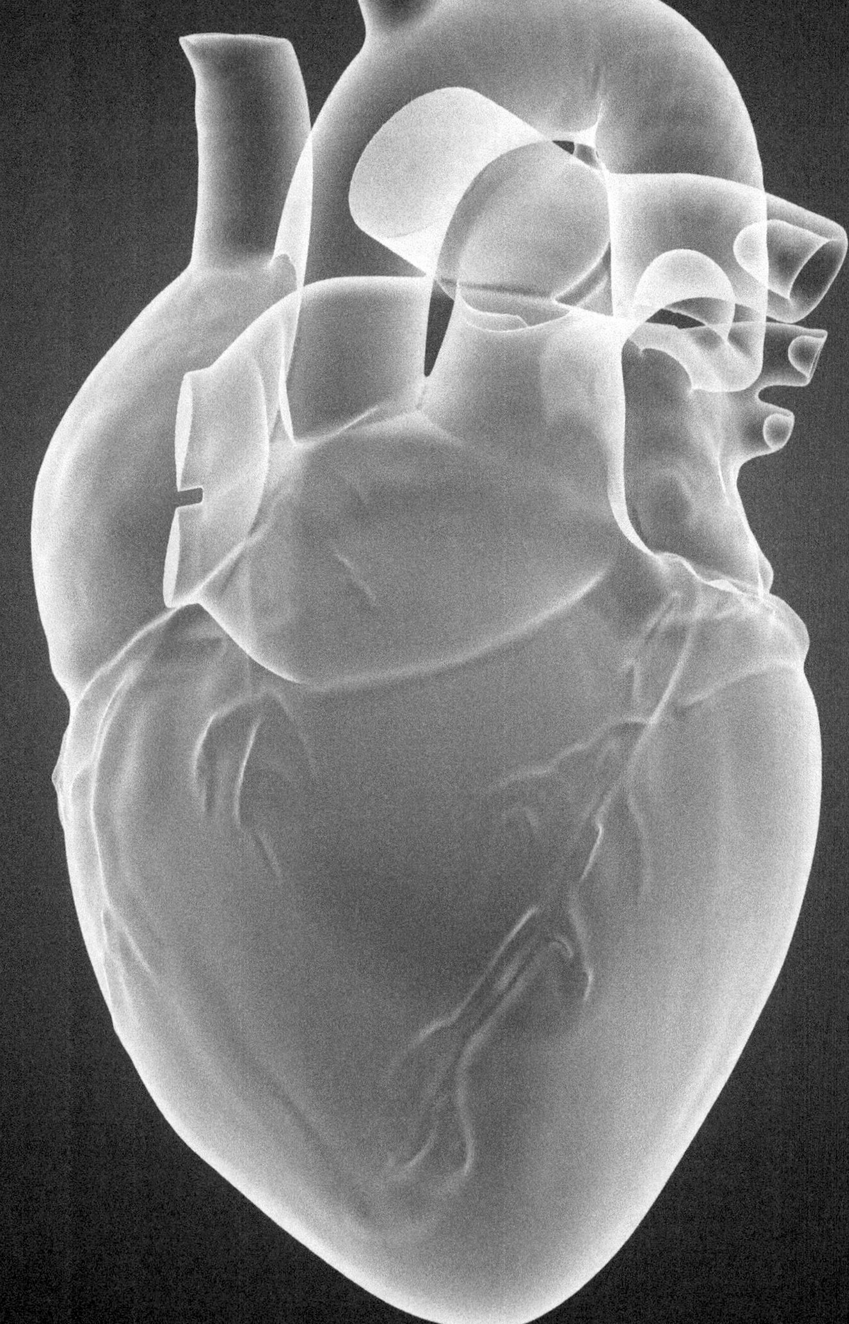
Part V.   A Heart Floating Among Styrofoam Planets

THE DUNKING GAME

Pretend to draw an arrow from a quiver
then aim at your favorite nine-year-old nephew.
Call it the *Robin Hood Dunk,* as he melts
into the blue. Then the no-hands *Evil Eye Dunk*
to the command "Do it again! Do it again!"
Then the *St. Valentine's Day Massacre Dunk.*
The Grand Slam Dunk. Poison Apple Dunk.
The Volleyball, Hot Cherry Pie, Grazing Cattle,
Slam-a Jama Hoopster, Secret Potion Dunks.
The Magic Wand, Arm Wrestle, Pinky Finger,
Dracula, Sniper Shot, Bore a Tall Blonde
to Death Dunks. The Puff of Sleeping Gas
from the Opened Book Dunk. Never once
thinking of dunking the way you were dunked,
The *Mean Older Boy Dunk,* head held under,
all fun drowned in the frantic struggle.
81 different dunks on Sunday afternoons
at Rehm Public Pool, cousin Tommy in a lifeguard chair,
Uncle Donald under the chair for "horseplay."
You dunked each other, striving to out-strangeify
before the *Off to College Dunk. The Return*
Home with a Man's Body and a Beard Dunk.
The Girlfriends, Apartments, Don't Say Hello,
Leave Abruptly, Imaginary Phone Call Dunks.
The I Need a Loan for a Car Dunk.
The Erasure of the Role of the Uncle Dunk.
The Hardly Know Each Other Dunk.
But you habituate to every repeat stimulus like
entering a cold pool. The initial flinch.
The clench of teeth, mouth retracted
in a painful grin. Then out of the blue,
the *Newborn Minnie May Hudson Dunk.*
The Dutiful Blood Relative, Show Up to the Church
and Don't Leave Early Dunk. The Meet at Midnight
at the Gossage Grill for Coffee Dunk.
The Baptism of Powdered Donuts Dunk.
Two Bobbing Heads at the Counter Dunk.

 Phillip J. Cozzi

WORDS THAT REFUSE TO LEAVE

When Aunt Clelia visited,
I learned the word *meatball*
refers to a human being.
I learned *gobbledygook, mangia,*
spumoni, stunade, Salerno,
greaseball, whop, dirtybastard.
Sitting beneath the kitchen table,
I learned the word *gnarled*
just by looking at her feet,
studied Mediterranean-colored
varicosities so beautifully scarred.
Drickydrock. Pasta and *fazul,*
because when Aunt Clelia sat down,
as if she would never rise again,
the world eased to a stop
and when Aunt Clelia spoke
cannoli held their breath
and words huddled around me
like Italian immigrants, hungry
newfound aunts and uncles.
Mannicoti. Pisane. Chewch.
No monster, but mobster.
No baseball cap, but fedora.
Spagette and the sovereign
olcountry. When I leapt
from under the table, like a gangster
from a birthday cake, I learned *Mafioso!*
is laughed with pride, all the while
my silent Irish mother stirred
a big pot of *sonofabitch.*

LASAGNA

It helped a lot to make lasagna while Anita was dying. Noodles-sauce-noodles-sauce- cheese-noodles-sauce-cheese-noodles-cheese. Just getting out of the bedroom. Focusing on fennel and cumulus tufts of ricotta over a red Florentine sea brought to mind the 6 Italian masterpieces you must see before you die. *The Arch of Constantine.* Venus, born daily on the walls of the Uffizi. The *David* must have worked up quite an appetite. *The Last Supper,* but Anita wasn't hungry. She lay Botticellian under layers and layers of quilts which her prayer group made, a dying art, as if perfecting the artof dying, nose tilted upward sniffing an aroma. We followed the recipe. Play-school-work-love-work-play-love-work-play-love, painting broad strokes of marinara with the back of a spoon. How heavy the scalding pan, hustled from oven to table, landed with a thud like consequence. Burnt edges of cheese rivaled the tenderness of lovers in Francisco Hayez's *The Kiss* and slaked a hunger for mercy. At 53, she perished in her Middle Ages. In 1622, Gian Lorenzo Bernini began the final masterwork, *Apollo e Dafne,* a pagan myth, capturing the exact moment her hand became leaves. Lasagna became persuasion. Anita became hope. As always, she died as soon as we left. By the time we got back, her forehead was cold against the lips and we prayed for her personal renaissance, *Rinascimento,* which in Italian means rebirth.

ANNIVERSARY DATE, WITH ORANGE MARMALADE

How not to think of him
        during this "Las Vegas-Style Show in Wisconsin"
before the woman is sawed in half,

before the bachelorette party is dragged on stage,
    rope tricks, levitations, corny jokes
told lovingly. This evening, I witness a man

put his head into the blades of a fan,
        wave to the audience and give warning
that we will not be able to sleep.

Passing Milk-Duds down to our twenty-something sons
    who salivate in the third row
while a barely clad assistant is folded

into a shoebox, only to reappear on motorcycle
        from stage left, I learn Houdini's wife
wrapped him in chains, in a crate,

and dropped him in a tank. I believe,
    as if tricked into being American,
that escaping death is what we do.

Wholesome families, from as far away as Indiana,
    indulge in the pleasure of this myth
to the throb of classic rock,

while hormone-deranged teens fiddle tongue dumbbells,
        toddlers squirm from mothers,
and dads' laser eyeballs track gyrations so obscene

they seem out of place in middle America.
        But who is not seduced by kitsch,
oldies, grunge, bedraggled diners with tiny tubs

of jellies in every flavor including orange marmalade,
     the globular shape and heft
of maple syrup dispensers. Our vows,

youthful deceptions which somehow became true,
  were conjured out of thin air,
not the magician's sentimental art

shouting bad taste, sophomorics on stage,
  but love's lasting illusion
never fully understood. The grand finale:

a helicopter appears out of nowhere
    in this tiny theatre in a strip mall
outside Lake Geneva. We are stunned

into silence by the reminder that life hovers
    between the real and the pretended. The truth is
the only time I rode on a helicopter was to harvest

an organ from San Antonio, Texas.
    He gave of himself to another.
Not a heart, but a liver.

A big, floppy, maroon mess of iron and tissue.
    As the curtain falls, we leap in applause
at the death-defying feat, still puzzling

"How did he do it?" How not
    to think of him who, after 31 years
of marriage, still teaches us something about love.

LOST EARRING

Just as we pulled up to the marquee, she sensed
absence, tugged one lobe then the other,
padded clothing, ran hand between car seats,
asked my help, believing two is always better
than one. Her face: a printed puzzle
to be studied to see what's missing:
a bauble valued only as a pair, a post
with dreamcatcher from which hung two link chains,
delicate but edgy, the look she was going for,
one hazel bead to make eyes sparkle. She reminded
they were given as a gift by me, although
I had no recollection, but did recall
at that moment my cousin Ruby who favored
large hoops and whose husband left Illinois
for California because he "wanted
to live by the ocean" and I thought
of my dad, eight years a widower, who
cannot comprehend why mom had to go
and why I have to go every time I leave him
to his caregiver. My wife in profile tilted her chin
into the air the way one does
when removing the clasp from an earring
or waiting for a kiss, then placed
the remaining earring in the cup holder between us,
awaiting its partner's return, while the missing earring,
the prodigal which pierced flesh and fled,
opened to me the bare and cinematic neckline.

A ROMANCE FOR CUTE

Nobody likes cute anymore
this synonym for vapid
barely attractive, an insult
as "Isn't that cute?"
a hypothetical in sarcasm
but if you'd seen
my three-year old son
in lime green trunks
hesitate at the edge
should he, shouldn't he
oversized swim goggles gripping
his crew-cutted ant head
then throw arms high
knees bent, enter air
lunge into summer, exchanging
one blue for another
find air again, guppy-mouthed
roleplay the Devonian Period
300 million years ago
and scramble four legged
from water to land
I might convince you
that cute beats edgy
that cute beats cool
smart sharp pop melodramatic
and even beats hip
that pinnacle of evolution
and synonym for hindquarters.

MUDBALL

Stepping by little continents hidden
on the untended, despised side of the house,
I fight the urge to pry one loose
and let it fly, or even better, after rain,
with mud molded into a ball
to throw at a telephone pole or fence post.
My meteors, like eyeless poets,
rarely hit the mark, but it was fun
filling summers between the ages five
and ten. Swim trunks or cut offs?
Trying to make just about anything
into a ball, larger than a meatball,
smaller than a baseball, just right
for a seven-year old hand. When
the pool day ended, we rolled our trunks
into towels. When summer ended,
we rolled that season into the next.
We made balls of different ages,
then friend groups, then whole decades
of our lives, marriages, parents, children,
clustered like memories, tin cup, water,
drinking air still and high through miles
of blue the night-beautiful universe,
molded partly musical, partly practical,
a reckless remembering of foxtail
and cattails, mountain ash and the ashes
of my sister-in-law, a pair of old boots.
What great packing this mudball made:
organic fragment of Pleistoceine plant
and microscopic organisms of today

in circular agreement, this overlooked miracle,
best removed from dirty hands
by scrubbing and scrubbing with Lava soap.
Grief, too, had the consistency of clay
especially when moiled with lantern light,
grit and prayer, a sudden, sodden concoction

Phillip J. Cozzi 93

only a child on hands and knees
could create, soft palms to polish,
then rise, little lithe arm at the ready,
eyes scanning the horizon for a target.

SCIENCE FAIR

My sixth-grade science teacher, Mrs. Galligan,
suggested we study what we love.
Joseph studied friction. Gabriella studied sugar.
Francesca studied whispering, proved
even the softest voices can be heard.
I studied crystals, particularly
the rhomboid blue copper sulfate crystal
by dangling in the solution a knotted string.
The seed, nucleus, nidus. I could have studied
a grain of sand, but the color was wrong.
I could have studied the frog leg,
but the copper solution was elemental
as sky in a jar. A crystal on a string
but growing, a crystal the shape of a story
that found in its growth a sense of time.
"Oh, I'll ask Kelvin, but just so you know…"
was Mrs. Galligan's way of suggesting
we study what we love, growing
spiky as bedhead on grammar school boy,
a prayer which gestated in a shoe box,
until the day I stood before God,
the judges, arms at my side,
straight as thermometer, at the folding table
altar in Monsignor Plunkett Hall,
my blood rising like a bicarbonate volcano
and my heart floating among Styrofoam planets.

ARROWS AND HANDS

I roused my sleeping man-child off the sofa
to go to bed, handed him his gym shoes
and suggested he brush his expensively-straightened teeth.

He stood for a long moment as if in trance,
an apparition, neither asleep nor wake, and in violation
of natural and scientific law, he mumbled

almost inaudibly, "Goodnight, Dad,"
as if one I have loved and lost
had risen, a metamorphosis, a vapor

from the forge of animal instinct, a fable
in human skin and garb, born of an age
more savage than temper, a pair of scales

held aloft, as the stars took possession
of the sky, as the arrows and the hands worthy
of them settled, as the ox slept eyes-open

while standing at the plough and the slumbering seeds
of things throughout the world poked green leaf
into night and perpetual Spring. He waited

with head bent, this symbol of magnanimous endurance
of unmerited suffering, for a goodnight hug.
Twenty years vaporized and whatever hidden from view

was imagined more beautiful still. His tousled hair
became spears of ripened grain, and his long
and long-held torso tender bark, swaying.

CHICKEN DRIPPINGS

During the next four hours, you are free
to make Francesca's birthday cake,
chill the sparkling cider, play ping pong
with her boyfriend Matt, admire Dar's backside
so nicely framed by apron strings.

Preheat oven to 400° and rub a fourth chicken
with unsalted butter under the skin
and in the cavity, then roast until caramelized
and the butter is brown. Strain
the buttery chicken drippings and reserve.

Try unsuccessfully to open a jar of whatever
ask Matt's help, and when he fails, give up,
run the jar under hot water, fail again
then acquiesce to Darlene's advice
and break the seal with a can opener.

Add the roasted chicken to the strained stock.
Bring to a rolling boil. Allow to reduce,
skimming the foam from the surface until only
a cup remains, until the liquid
is thick enough to coat a spoon, until
it tastes like family memory.

Setting the table with maple leaf napkin holders
acknowledges the annual diminution
of birthdays, while inventing the truth
of birthdays, like living an unwritten memoir
of a young woman repossessing her life.

Pour the liquid through a fine mesh strainer.
Add the reserved buttery chicken drippings.
Stir in 2 tablespoons finely diced shallot,
then parsley, tarragon and minced fresh chervil.
Hold hands at table for a moment, this distillation
of a year, an extract of four lives filling the air.

ODE TO THE OTHER SIDE

In Frankenstein's bathroom, as it was known
to my seven siblings, was a rusted cabinet

with a mirrored front. On the other side
of that mirror, a coppery rash

bubbled in blisters, an impetigo
from thousands of showers. But peacock green

appeared in tiny wisps and purpura presented
alternative beauty, like the other side

of a smile or impossibility or family life
or the untended side of a home.

The other side of broken. The other
side of silence, uncertainty, mother,

father. The other side of obsession
in scrutiny of blemish or bangs.

The other side of shadow, song
and the other side of although.

The other side of giggling heard
from the other side of a bedroom wall.

The other side of ordinary, oblique,
an octave or angle. The other side

of any child's school day morn
to marvel at one's monstrous self

in the mirror of a yellow-white cabinet
over the sink in Frankenstein's bath.

TALKING TRASH

Like glaciers, pieces of cracked cement slab shift
      imperceptibly making odd-shaped continents by the garbage cans
on the apron behind my parents' bungalow. Once, epic wars raged
      on this triangular basketball court. An early crack, the free-throw line.
Now, the ghosts of Bobby Stopka, gone to ALS, and Les Stromberg,
      gone to heroin, pick teams and we go to it with an invisible ball:
head fakes, behind-the-back passes, low crossovers, and held follow through
      as 18-foot jumpers kiss off the boards. The dead remember
to pick and roll, fill the spaces, box out, look away, lean in,
      bend the knees and cut off the baseline. The dead have attitude.
Pale blue butterwort, wildflower left in the wake of the great thaw,
      taunts from the cracks, "Show me what you're made of,
                    Grandma" and "All day, baby."

CHURCHES

Tiny volume of a tear, crimson discoid blood cells slipping through capillaries, cereal box, the pelvic cup where prayer gestates, beneath a grand piano on Christmas morning, Sunday shoes with toes in the front pew, ceramic vase filled with the stems of buffoonish Dogbane, the steamy backseat of a policecruiser parked in the most remote spot behind The Fire Bell Pub, the pearls of Cassiopeia, an oval pendant on the forehead, atrium of a cobalt eye, crystal breath on a winter morning. Never the shortest distance between two points. Never a stain, but certainly a cube of ice floating amid fizz of cherry cola, or the waxy movie theatre cup praying for a refill. Never a photo of the smiling face of an aunt taped to a refrigerator but the refrigerator itself, the dome of the liver, the tremulous parcel of air carrying Johnny Come Down to Hilo, Italy, abandoned merchant vessel, the prison cell of the poet Etheridge Knight, space beneath waterfall or ironing board, teepee, coffee pot, hollow center of plum seed, tackle box, iron stove, supraclavicular fossa, lone shepherd's cottage, a red pasture at dusk, a barn after birthing, or the covered passageway filled with crisp leaves beside the cellar door, tool shed, navel, boxcar, the hollow behind the knee, pup tent, mausoleum, and when I drive past the steeples, stained glass and women skilled at smiling through malice, I realize I'd rather lay curled, naked, shivering, holy in the sanctuary of garbage can, kitten's ear, game closet, sugar cone.

THE GOOD EXHAUSTION

of making 400 empanadas after midnight, two-stepping dance marathon, turning soil and spreading mulch, hefting a dresser to the third-floor walkup, performing CPR or portage, cleaning up after Sunday dinner, building the backyard ice rink, pulling out tree stumps. Not rationalizing with a demented person. Not the constant tiresome display of sexual availability. Not the tedium of coffeehouse conversation but carrying the sacks of coffee beans that have been out all night in the rain, the heavy lifting of earning trust, the 36-hour caregiver's day, befriending the unlovable, the ancestral labor of pulling Conestoga across the divide. After rage or the fourth quarter of a full-court BBall game with nobody on the bench. And I think of Mr. Thomas, a simple man, father to my best friend Mikey, pipe-fitter unskilled in the trade of beautiful lies. He spent his days beneath the streets as if cleaning moral sewer. I never heard him speak but know he knew at deflation of day that head-to-pillow, sleep-of-death, lasting joy of exhaustion.

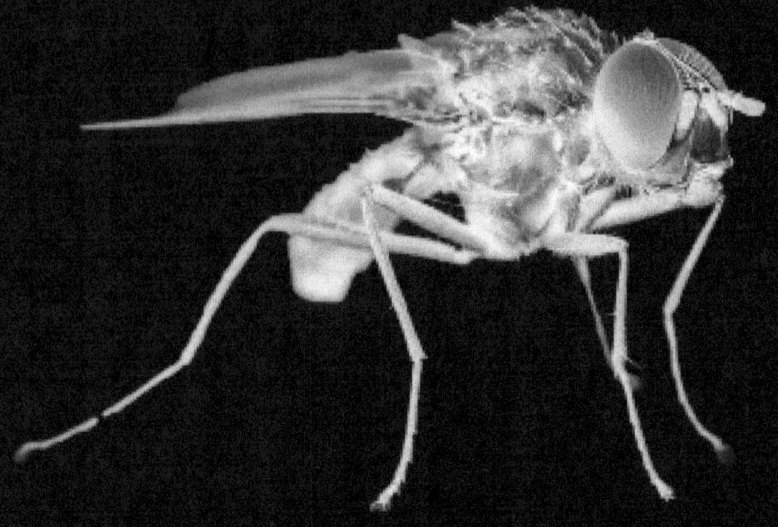

Part VI. Unworldly Pilot and Navigator Charting the Metaphysical

ARS POETICA with a FRUIT FLY

We read poetry together in bed last night.
I held the book while this crazed aviator
hurled her winged wholeness at the booklight,
frantic for insight, optimistic Drosophila,
Icarus, Don Quixote, impatient angel,
my Lindbergh circling the Eiffel
then lighting biplane down on the runway
of W.H. Auden's poem, after long flight,
also paying respects to W.B. Yeats,
in memorium. She performed interpretive dance
right there on print, more crazed than solemn,
then took to air, barnstorming
the final stanza like circus bleachers,
swooping up to write in cursive all
which can be said regarding flight.
My wind walker, unworldly pilot
and navigator charting metaphysical.
A travel companion approaching
a twinkling city grid of words at night.
Challenge, triumph, twin and muse
veering into more compelling air.
Goodnight, my darling, a thousand thanks
for all your kindnesses, each syllable
a pulse from the world's tiniest heart.

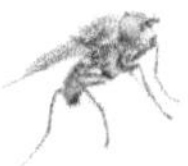

Phillip J. Cozzi 103

PINE CREEK
(After Sasha Khan)

Everything I once thought was important,
the grades, the girls, the basketball games,
I know now as irrelevant

nonsense, blather, on which I oughtn't
to have idled years. But summer days,
long ago, when everything was so important,

meeting Sasha, the 4th of July, the scent
of Pine Creek, Montana, the campfire flames,
I know now as irrelevant,

glowed with permanence. How the now non-existent
buffalo herd which escaped one school day,
when every living thing was so important,

and we huddled in the back of a restaurant
where Mrs. Hjertsen taught us how to dance,
the gist of which is now irrelevant,

but in that moment, crucial was the hand
in hand, cautious was the hand on waist,
for who's to say what truly is important?
Who knew then to love the irrelevant?

WHY I LOVE PICKLES

Because my sister Lizzie loved pickles,
    large green crunchy cold ones
    you had to grip with a fist
    and extend your chin far forward
    so that pickle juice did not run
    down your neck to your shirt,
    preferring those bumpy as Darwin's toad
    and usually snatched from a jar
    so big it took an entire length
    of arm, right to the shoulder,
    to get the one you wanted
    best gobbled between sack races
    and the water balloon toss, barefoot.

Because the Kearn boys threw that kitten,
    a black Maine Coone with white breast
    and one white front paw, on the roof
    of their garage, then pitched crab apples
    to make it jump down, my sister Lizzie
    kept that kitten in a shoebox.

Because that cat grew to be King
    of the Alley, enormous, fearless
    and feared by neighborhood dogs,
    returned each night bloody as a prize-fighter
    after one more round of ripped flesh
    cracked bone, chewed ear, survival,
    and because that cat got so sick
    I could lift him into the carrier
    without a fight and because mom and dad
    both worked, I took the cat,
    alone as a 10 year old, to the vet
    who told me it would cost less
    to put him to sleep than treat him,
    fearing my dad's anger at the expense.

Because in later years he began to look

like Winston Churchill, defender of liberal democracy,
maintaining centrality of presence,
even splitting allegiances
as a practical sociologist
knowing who to snugglerub
for the Friskies Party Mix with ocean whitefish
and flavors of shrimp, crab and tuna,
then rhapsodizing in his excesses,
fattening, could no longer groom,
grew mats of hair which
had to be cut off with scissors,
dragged his hind legs
and finally wiped himself on kitchen linoleum.

Because Pickles survived
    that vet visit another 20 years,
    a great companion to our mother
    long after Lizzie and I strayed away.

Because of his posthumous ascension,
    he remained a contemporary figure
    of extraordinary influence
    over we who remained obsessed
    not only with the cat
    but how he viewed us.

SONNET to the DOG EARRED PAGE

Bless the papery auricle which listens
for the body entering the pages
of bedsheet, reminds how far we've come,
how far we have yet to go
and helps the literary omnivore find
their place in any novel
habitat. The little flap flags
favorite poems, the ones with teeth
for tearing flesh, teeth for grinding seed,
ones to which we return like tongue.
And when the eyelid blinds are drawing
down, we make a new animal
origami with a single crease, pinna
of our guide dog into night.

VIBURNUM

A darling cemetery, perfectly ungroomed,
right on the way to the train station,
reminds you not to work so hard and you can't help,

no matter how briskly you walk,
but read the rain-battered sandstones
and, with a little quick math, calculate the age at death.

Angela Haas, 1889 – 1894,
and Michele Haas, 1890 – 1897,
have markers overgrown by the flowering shrub, viburnum.

Linneaus in Species Planetarum
devised a Latin binomial system
so that every plant also gets a first and last name,

such as *Viburnum dentatum,*
humble arrowwood with glabrous buds,
but shrubs have no souls, no joy, no acceptance,

no ability to rise and walk,
cannot fulfill themselves,
nor glory in the knowledge of dallying cloudlets.

Low branches feel around
in the morning darkness. Grave stones tilt
together like human head. What good can you do the sisters now

while boarding the impatient train,
but imagine the errors at piano,
the shirked chores, the unbreakable bond and the tiny
pink and white flowers which would have blossomed under their touch?

VIRGINIA AND ALLEN

Virginia Knotweed is not your high school librarian
but a shrub. Diminutive, delicate buds,
fused the length of twinned stems,
come into focus only with the magnifying glass,
tiny pink helmets and shoulder pads,
and bring to mind Allen Ross,
footballer friend at Fenwick Boys Preparatory,
who vomited out the principal's window,
left college, married, divorced and disappeared.
He destroyed a LazyBoy by flexing his deltoids,
bursting the sides out with his elbows.
No one was more admired or hated.
No girl could resist. Striking, with black hair.
Rumored to have thrown himself off a windmill.
Only after close inspection can you see
hundreds of tiny pink Allens waiting to burst
into the emptiness he wanted. Prodigies,
on the way out. Virginia offers a sprig –
not the ancient truth that youthful promise
droops under the weight of its own flowerhead -
but this insistent weed which God has woven
out of boredom and now endures
on its own frailty. The soft brown eyes
of two coneflowers, which have lost their petals,
gaze upward like an adoring fiancé.

HONG KONG CRANE

After H.W. Leung

                        How
                   privileged
                to have known
              you, if only briefly,
            skyping from your
              island home. Not
              bad privilege
                of which
              I am both
                accused and
                  guilty. But
              the good kind,
                  that of having
                    been a lodger
                  in my mother,
                    from comma to
                      paragraph,
                    of positing
                    paired femurs,
                    chambers of
                    the heart, to
                    be vertebrate,
                  mammal and
                  mortal, and if
            one day, our poet-farmer,
          your gaze lifts from swampy gallery
        to find a crane, beak-tipped, across a shallow
    pond as if standing in portrait, may your artist's soul
      migrate toward a view with two focal points,
      us and them, sketch a horizontal line, trace words of
    grass to occupy the foreground, light washing water,
      and tranquility alight as in a moment
    of acceptance of guilt. The perspective of
    sky to land is as significant as the sense
    of scale: a view from a cluster of
    cells clinging to endometrium, the
      gender   of a poem,
      the   flight
      of   text,
                                b
                                a
                                l
                                a
                                n
                                c
                                e
of colors compressed toward horizon, a true realization of the rare privilege that is ours.

 Phillip J. Cozzi

BRIEF ACQUAINTANCE AT THE LURIE GARDENS

Most of us want to die at home, with family and without pain
but I admire your Trumanesque power of decision
having chosen this sidewalk, shaded in the irony
of the arborvitae, tree of life. Fetal fingers,
neither leaf nor needle, extend a handful
of still-green baby pine cones, each offering
exactly eight seeds. Oversized trash receptacles
eye me suspiciously, like docents, as I lean in
to discern your facial expression. Can't tell
 if you died at peace, but you should have.
Gray brown except for the black toupee,
blonde fuzz on the ass, and a taste of mustard
on the fuselage. Each shaped like Lake Michigan,
your wings tremble in the breeze, wind urging
post-mortem flight, a daughter's invisible hand
nudging "Wake up! Wake up!" Still,
you are blind as soil and soon to be.
Your face is nondescript, as if specifically designed
to escape notice, and your life, I guess,
was not the stuff of film noir. Your nose
was never flattened by a rifle butt,
and you never escaped Russia in a pickle barrel.
Had you been mugging silly faces with your sisters
in the home, junior accountants in your cells?
Did you die defending the hive
from yellow-jackets? The sting of failure?
Or die of takotsubo's, the broken heart syndrome,
while your larvae were eaten with shredded coconut,
 wrapped in banana leaves and steamed?
Had you just returned from vacation
and realized there was no pollen in the refrigerator?
The truth is darker. Winston Churchill yawns
in his villa at Potsdam, and my life,
like the General Eisenhower Expressway,
oscillates between smooth sailing and suffocation.
Of course, I have nothing with which to resuscitate,
except a pen and a volume of light literature,

Phillip J. Cozzi   111

The Banyard Street Tightrope Walker,
the back pages on which I scribble haphazard eulogy.
You were laid, flew and died but I
believe that in that moment of mating
or laying eggs you knew savage happiness.
The bouquets on these eastern cedars
tip toward each other like wine glasses

                              for your final toast.

 Phillip J. Cozzi

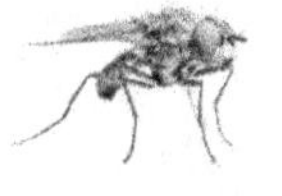

Phillip J. Cozzi 113

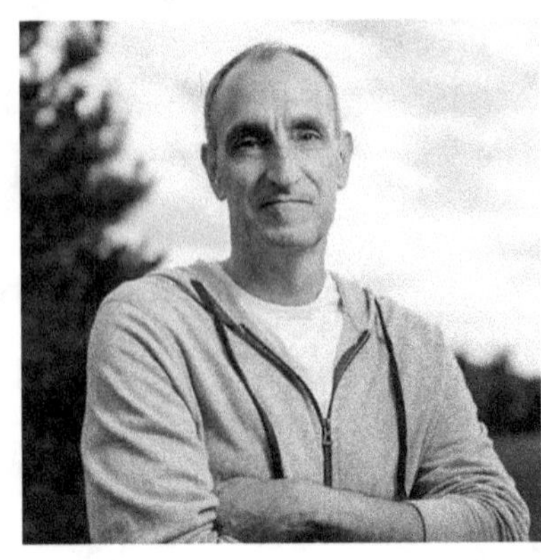

Phillip J. Cozzi, MD, attended University of Chicago Medical School, completed residency and chief medical residency at Northwestern Memorial Hospitals and fellowships in Pulmonary and Critical Care Medicine at the University of Chicago. He has served as Medical Director of Critical Care at Elmhurst Memorial Hospital for the past 25 years. Cozzi completed a Masters of Fine Arts in Writing at The School of The Art Institute of Chicago. His poems have appeared in *The New England Journal of Medicine, JAMA, The Annals of Internal Medicine, Rhino* and *The Southwest Review.* He has received the inaugural poetry prize from the American College of Physicians and the Morton Marr Poetry Prize from *The Southwest Review.* He is married to Dr. Darlene Cozzi and is the father of Gabriella, Francesca, Phillip and Joseph.

All author proceeds will be directed to a charity for Ukrainian relief.

ACKOWLEDGEMENTS

For their generous spirits, skill, encouragement, and for reviewing parts of this book, I wish to thank Amy England, Christian Campbell, Jesse Ball, Mary Cross, Nathan Hoks, Rosellen Brown and, especially, Elise Paschen, without whose unwavering support, kindness and lively imagination I would not have made it through the first three weeks of grad school. Only I can have a true appreciation of how Elise's aesthetic and editorial acumen has informed nearly each of these poems. Thanks also to Sally Alatalo for sharing her love of bookmaking.

For all my patients, for providing inspiration.

For my two most life-changing school teachers: Mr. Sean Concannon, who made learning so much fun that I did not want to stop, and Mr. James Kuchinski, who introduced me to literature.

For being my poetry pen pal, I thank John Van Peenan. For being a new-found friend in art, I thank Otto Rutt.

For my newfound friends at Gold Wake, Kyle and Paul, for their selfless promotion and defense of the arts.

For their love and sparkling wit, I thank my siblings Larry, Nancy, Lizzie, Barbara, Peggy, Bob and, especially, Paula, for teaching me the alphabet and how to use it.

For my children, Gabriella, Francesca, Phillip and Joseph, for providing wonder, happiness and confidence in the future. For always helping selflessly, especially with the design of this book, special thanks to Phillip.

For my wife, Darlene, who makes each day more beautiful.

 Phillip J. Cozzi